Digital Welfare for the Th

This book is about the ways in which digital technology can contribute to the welfare of older people. The Internet, mobile phones and other technologies have changed how we live and work. Such technologies also shape how services for older people are organised in ways that potentially place carers and older people at the centre of service provision. Telecare can make homes 'smart' so that they are more comfortable and less risky for people who can take advantage of devices that help make them independent members of their community.

Digital welfare is part of the broader project in Britain and elsewhere to adopt new information and communications technologies (ICTs) to organise and deliver health and social welfare services. This includes mundane technologies such as an alarm to call for help to complex telecare 'smart homes' and electronic patient records. The intended and unintended consequences of such new technologies must be explored if we are to benefit from these innovations. Based on recent research, this book seeks to highlight and examine the new opportunities and dilemmas that confront older people and all those concerned with their welfare in the network society.

This edited collection provides original contributions from leading academics and researchers in the field to access the evidence for improved professional integration and user-centred health and social care services for older people arising from health informatics. *Digital Welfare for the Third Age* will be of interest to all those working with older people.

Brian D. Loader is Co-Director of the Social Informatics Research Unit, Department of Sociology, University of York.

Michael Hardey is Reader in Sociology at the Hull/York Medical School and the Department of Social Sciences at the University of Hull.

Leigh Keeble is a Development Officer in local government, and previously a Research Fellow at the University of York.

Digital Welfare for the Third Age

Health and social care informatics for older people

Edited by
Brian D. Loader, Michael Hardey
and Leigh Keeble

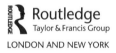

LONDON AND NEW YORK

First published 2009
by Routledge
2 Park Square, Milton Park, Abingdon, Oxon OX14 4RN

Simultaneously published in the USA and Canada
by Routledge
270 Madison Avenue, New York, NY 10016

Routledge is an imprint of the Taylor & Francis Group, an informa business

© 2009 selection and editorial matter, Brian D. Loader, Michael Hardey and
Leigh Keeble; individual chapters, the contributors

Typeset in Sabon by Taylor & Francis Books
Printed and bound in Great Britain by
TJ International Ltd, Padstow, Cornwall

British Library Cataloguing in Publication Data
A catalogue record for this book is available from the British Library

Library of Congress Cataloging in Publication Data
Digital welfare for the third age : health and social care informatics for older
people / edited by Brian D. Loader, Michael Hardey, and Leigh Keeble.
       p. ; cm.
    Includes bibliographical references.
    1. Medical telematics. 2. Geriatrics–Data processing. 3. Older people–
Services for. I. Loader, Brian, 1958- II. Hardey, Michael. III. Keeble, Leigh.
    [DNLM: 1. Telemedicine. 2. Aged. 3. Health Services for the Aged. 4.
Information Systems. 5. Internet. 6. Self-Help Devices. WT 26.5 D574 2009]
    R119.95D54 2009
    025.06′61–dc22
                        2008023709

ISBN10: 0-415-45408-5 (hbk)
ISBN10: 0-415-45409-3 (pbk)
ISBN10: 0-203-88653-4 (ebk)

ISBN13: 978-0-415-45408-7 (hbk)
ISBN13: 978-0-415-45409-4 (pbk)
ISBN13: 978-0-203-88653-3 (ebk)

Contents

Illustrations

Tables

Figures

Box

Contributors

Sue Baines is Reader in Social Policy in the Research Institute for Health and Social Change at Manchester Metropolitan University (MMU). Sue joined MMU in summer 2007. Prior to that, she was a principal researcher working in the Institute for Policy and Practice at Newcastle University. She has many years' experience of working in multidisciplinary research environments to deliver applied social research. She has managed projects from sponsors including the Economic and Social Research Council (ESRC), the Joseph Rowntree Foundation, the Department of Communities and Local Government, and Arts Council England. Sue has published widely on aspects of small enterprise, social inclusion, livelihoods and unpaid work.

Sue came to academia as a doctoral student in CURDS (Centre for Urban and Regional Development Studies) at Newcastle University under the auspices of PICT (Programme on Information and Communication Technologies). She completed an ESRC post-doctoral fellowship in 1999 which examined the experiences of employees who turned to self-employment during the restructuring of the UK print and broadcast media. Since then, she has undertaken studies of marginal self-employment, creative livelihoods and, more recently, volunteering. She joined the Social and Business Informatics (SBI) team at Newcastle University Business School in 2003 to take on the role of managing the evaluation component of a national e-government project known as FAME (Framework for Multi-Agency Environments). She has an ongoing interest in public services and their continued reliance on unpaid work (within and beyond the household). Her particular interest within this domain is in the increasingly prominent role of the third sector in public policy and service delivery. See http://www.mmucfe.co.uk/people/drsusanbaines/.

Julienne Hanson is Professor of House Form and Culture at the Bartlett, University College London, where she has been a teacher and researcher since 1975. Her research has included profiling the UK's housing stock with the needs of older people in mind, investigating the layout and design of residential care homes in relation to quality of life issues and studying the housing, support and care needs of both older people with visual impairments and the housing and support needs of people of working age with impaired sight. She has recently completed research into mainstreaming 'telecare' services in the homes of older people, remodelling sheltered housing and residential care homes to extra care housing and ways of designing the public open spaces of residential areas so as to minimise antisocial behaviour.

Michael Hardey is Reader in Sociology at the Hull/York Medical School based at the Universities of Hull and York and is a member of the Department of Social Sciences at the University of Hull. His work includes seeking to understand the role of the Internet as part of e-health and, more broadly, on the mediation of relationships. Recently, he has studied the nature of Web 2.0 and the way it may change the engagement of users with professionals and information about health.

Elizabeth Johnson Avery is an Assistant Professor in Advertising and Public Relations at the University of Tennessee. Her research utilises both persuasion and public opinion theory to enhance public relations practice and research, specifically in political and health campaign contexts. Her work has been published in major journals such as *Public Relations Review*, *Journal of Public Relations Research*, *Public Relations Journal* and *Health Communication*.

Leigh Keeble was a Translational Research Fellow on the e-Society programme at the University of York. She was the researcher on the Department of Health-funded project 'Wired for the Third Age?' with Brian Loader and Mike Hardey. She currently works in local government.

Brian D. Loader is Co-Director of the Social Informatics Research Unit (SIRU) based at the University of York, UK. His academic interests are focused around the emergence of new information and communications technologies (ICTs), such as the Internet, the social, political and economic factors shaping their development and diffusion and their implications for social, economic, governmental and cultural change. He is General Editor of the international journal *Information, Communication & Society* and has published extensively in this field.

Wendy Macias is an Associate Professor in Advertising and Public Relations at the University of Georgia. Her research focuses on consumer behaviour issues related to interactive advertising, direct-to-consumer pharmaceutical advertising and online health communication. She has published her research in journals such as the *Journal of Advertising*, *Health Communication*, *Journal of Health Communication* and *Health Marketing Quarterly*.

Sally J. McMillan is an Associate Professor in Advertising and Public Relations at the University of Tennessee. Her research focuses on exploring interactivity, definitions and history of new media, online research methods, health communication and the impact of communication technology on society. She has published in journals such as *Journal of Advertising, Health Communication, Journal of Health Communication,* and *New Media and Society.*

Dorota Osipovič is a PhD student at the School of Slavonic and East European Studies, University College London. She has an MA in Sociology from Warsaw University. She has participated in a number of research projects looking into migration and citizenship issues, the support needs of people with vision impairment and social aspects of lifestyle monitoring technologies.

John Percival is an Associate Lecturer in Health and Social Care at the Open University, a Research Fellow in Social and Policy Sciences at the University of Bath, an independent research consultant and part-time social worker. John has previously worked as a Research Fellow at University College London and at the University of Bristol, where his predominantly qualitative research included projects that examined older people's housing aspirations, the impact of sight loss on social exclusion and lay and professional perspectives on telecare service development.

John's main research interests focus on the relationship between housing, health and social care needs; the emotional, psychological and practical implications of sight loss; technology and health monitoring in the homes of people with disabilities; and qualitative research as a policy and practice tool.

John is currently working on a number of projects that examine the contribution of assistive technologies to the well-being of people with sight loss who live in supported housing. John is also researching end of life care in nursing homes and care homes.

John Powell is Associate Clinical Professor of Epidemiology and Public Health at the University of Warwick. His first degree was in Social and Political Sciences, before he gained a medical degree and worked as a doctor in the NHS for 10 years. Since undertaking a PhD investigating information needs and the use of the Internet in the area of mental health care, he has become a full-time researcher in the area of e-Health. His particular focus is on the use of information and communication technologies to improve public health.

Darren Reed's research interests are in the area of ethnomethodology (EM), conversation analysis (CA), reflexivity and Internet communication. His PhD was an ethnomethodological analysis of 'newsgroup' interaction that used the analysis to reflect back on the conceptual foundations of EM and CA.

Over the past few years, Darren has looked to combine Science and Technology Studies and Human Computer Interaction and has split his time between Sociology, Psychology and Computer Science. His interests include mundane interaction with technologies in broad social contexts that incorporate people's histories, experiences and expectations.

Darren has been working in a variety of fields including:

- Inclusive design – an area interested in promoting the design of everyday technology devices that are attractive and can be used by older people.
- Transport management and information systems.
- Assistive technology, especially the development of commonplace technologies such as the telephone to support isolated elderly individuals.

Currently, he is interested in the use of social networking sites and virtual environments.

Andrew Webster is Professor in the Sociology of Science and Technology, Director of SATSU, Head of the Department of Sociology, University of York, national coordinator of the ESRC stem cells initiative and former director of the UK Innovative Health Technologies Programme. His most recent book is *Health, Technology and Society: A Sociological Critique*, Palgrave Macmillan, 2007.

Rob Wilson is a Senior Lecturer in Management at the Newcastle University Business School (NUBS) and a Deputy Director of the Centre for Knowledge, Innovation, Technology and Enterprise (KITE). Within KITE, he leads the Social and Business Informatics (SBI) group of five staff and four associates. See the KITE website at http://www.ncl.ac.uk/kite.

With over 10 years' experience working on and leading public sector information systems (IS) development and implementation projects, he has lectured widely on IS in public sector contexts to a range of audiences including policy makers, managers, practitioners, system suppliers and academics. He teaches on a range of undergraduate and postgraduate programmes with a particular interest in research methods. Rob's research interests are in public sector IS: the role that IS plays in organisational change and interorganisation partnership working.

His research career began in health informatics where he was heavily involved in a range of projects including e-prescribing (ETP and repeat prescribing) and decision support (PRODIGY) projects for the Department of Health (including decision support, patient records and messaging). Since joining the Business School in 2002, he has worked on a programme of projects tackling challenge partnership working and IS in a range of education, welfare, health and social care contexts (including children, young people and older adults), which has been a significant UK policy imperative since 1997. This work has been funded by a mixture of the European Commission (FP5 and FP6), government departments/agencies (DH, DCLG, NHS, GO-NE), local government and research councils (EPSRC, ESRC). Possibly the most significant project is the DCLG-funded Framework for Multi-agency Environments (FAME) project (see http://www.fame-uk.org/), which produced a range of tools to support public service partnerships to develop and improve multiagency working arrangements. His current work is largely focused on 'telecare' and includes a Framework 6 project called OLDES (http://www.oldes.eu/) looking at the development of 'tele-befriending' systems in Italy and the Czech Republic and a Department of Health ICT research project on Integrating Telecare where he runs a work package on Integrating Health and Social Care. See: http://www.ncl.ac.uk/nubs/staff/profile/rob.wilson.

Acknowledgements

The origins of this collection are to be found in a research project undertaken by the editors entitled *Wired for the Third Age* which was funded by the UK Department of Health under the auspices of its *Modernising Adult Social Care* programme. More specifically, the chapters were primarily developed from contributions to a small symposium organised to disseminate the research project findings that took place in the enchanting city of York. We would like to thank the participants who helped shape some of the ideas expressed in this book. We are also grateful for permission to include the chapter by Sally J. McMillan, Elizabeth Johnson Avery and Wendy Macias, which was first published recently in the journal *Information, Communication & Society*. Special thanks go to Sarah Shrive-Morrison for providing administrative support and encouragement. As ever, we are all in debt to the love and support of our respective spouses, children and colleagues and thank them all sincerely.

1 Introduction

*Michael Hardey, Brian D. Loader
and Leigh Keeble*

This book is about older people, their homes, technology and data.

In any area where a range of professions, practitioners, state and voluntary agencies combine with technologies that may include a device connected to the Internet and a switch connected to an alarm to deliver services to users, there is considerable scope for confusion and procrastination. Terminology such as health informatics, telecare, telehealth, assistive technology, telemedicine, e-health, telepsychiatry, smart homes, intelligent accommodation and so forth can be found scattered across the academic and policy literature. These categories reflect academic, practice and organisational differences as well as a tendency for the resulting specialism to develop a narrow focus around innovation and problem solving. Here, telecare will be used simply to refer to the broad range of devices, software and so forth that may be available to older people. Telemedicine enthusiasts have argued that it has 'the potential of having a greater impact on the future of medicine than any other modality' (DeBakey 1995: 3). In the light of medical developments since the 1990s, this claim appears rather exaggerated, but it denotes an underlying tendency to view new technology as central to the improvement of human health and sense of wellness. In addition, shades of technological determination, if not optimism, have left a legacy on the development of digital welfare.

Making connections between people, places and organisation

The delivery of health and social care in the UK has been transformed since the 1980s through a process of neoliberal marketisation with its emphasis upon consumerism, individual choice and responsibility. For older people and those with chronic illnesses, this challenged the tendency to view them as more or less passive recipients of care and medical expertise. Past notions of frailty highlight the construct of age and gender manifest in the label 'little old lady' (Arber & Ginn 1995). Social gerontologists remind us that people are 'aged by culture' as much as by ageing bodies (Gullette 2004). The publication, *Choosing Health: Making Healthy Choices Easier* (Department of Health 2004a), highlights a contemporary ideal-type service user in the guise of the informed consumer/citizen. This places information, in terms of both lived experience and abstract medical and other knowledge, at the centre of the delivery of care. In effect, older clients of health and social care are cast in the role of 'knowing users' of a coordinated system. This publication (Department of Health 2004a) frames the role of health and social services in terms of enabling individuals to generate their own health and well-being (Hughes 2004). Underlying structures of governance are visible here that reveal the New Labour project to forge a contractual relationship with individualised citizens (Fisher 2007). This has shaped a notion of informatisation that is predicated upon a seamless and systematic connection between different professional groups (e.g. doctors and social workers), different parts of the health and social care system (e.g. housing and social services) and different levels of government (national and local) across different geographical localities. In policy terms, the process also reflects a concern to write responsible users of public services into a pivotal role, so that they are seen as active agents in a health/care process rather than the object of intervention. Manifest in the Expert Patient programme outlined in *Saving Lives* (Department of Health 1999), those with chronic conditions are encouraged to engage in self-care and management while the state provides a menu of resources. A sense of empowerment can raise the self-esteem and quality of life for individuals as their embodied knowledge and experiences are placed at the centre of decision making that is shared with practitioners (Wilson 2001).This requires, as the NHS Information Authority (2004) puts it, that 'patient centred care' is the aim of the informatisation process. Congruent with such policies and practices, the informatisation process had to recognise the place of the service user as a partner with practitioners. Users had also to be recognised as participants within information systems instead of subjects to be represented in digital forms that potentially include x-ray images, patient records and assessments from social workers.

The national programme of computerising the health care system was initiated in the late 1990s when the NHS Executive set a target of 2005 for what was described as an 'electronic healthcare record' to be implemented across all Trusts (NHS Executive 1998). Previously, different parts of the health and social care system had made use of computerised records with varying degrees of complexity and success (e.g. The Wessex Regional Health Authority's much criticised implementation of IT (Beynon-Davies & Lloyd-Williams 1999)). Past practices in relation to information reflect divides between primary and secondary care as well as different territories that are mapped out in boundaries between national and local accountability and budgets. The Wanless (2002) review of NHS finance, *Securing our Future Health*, marked the commitment to invest in information technology at increased levels in the light of 'piecemeal and poorly integrated' systems that existed at the time. In theory, some £214 million of central government funds were to be spent between 1991 and 2001 on various informatisation projects, but much of this was expended in other areas. A new national programme that would contract out the work was announced in 2002. The English National Programme for IT (NPfIT) was coordinated by a team of consultants and implemented through strategic health authorities.

Large-scale government computer projects have a problematic history. The National Audit Office examined the progress made in delivering the informatisation of health and social care against the original plans and costs of the programme (National Audit Office 2006). While the Audit Office noted that there had been major progress, it also highlighted failure to meet a number of significant milestones. In particular, the local delivery of the first phases of the NHS Care Records Service and the advanced integrated IT systems has experienced a series of serious delays. Deployment of the National Clinical Record anticipated in December 2004 was only available in pilot form by late 2006. While the software for *Choose and Book* was delivered on time, the take-up of the system to support patient choice was markedly slower than initially planned. In addition, the Audit Office noted that there were concerns voiced by NHS staff as to exactly what the programme was trying to achieve, when systems would be delivered and what they would do. NPfIT has since become *Connecting for Health*, which has been described as the 'largest non military IT project attempted in the world' (Bowers 2007).

Social work practice has assumed the presence of clients in the same way that medical practice has made assumptions about the role of patients. The modernisation of health and social services has brought into being the service user as well as the notion of service providers. Webster (2002) argues that the introduction of technology can shift the 'medical repertoire' so that the concept of the 'patient' is changed (see Webster 2002: Ch. 5). As noted earlier, at a broader level, there has been a policy transformation that has had an impact on the practice of medicine and social work in terms of service users' position in the delivery of care. A consequence of this change is the development of inter-agency teams and the increasing role of partnership across professions (Glendinning *et al.* 2002). Despite changing terminology, the label 'client' or 'patient' remains in common currency among practitioners. However, rather than an individual, these categories should be seen as a relationship that is negotiated by all those involved. The 1996 Community Care (Direct Payments) Act was extended to older people in 2000 so that local authorities could provide cash in lieu of services (Glendinning *et al.* 2000). An older person may therefore become an employer of a care assistant as well as being seen as a patient by a general practitioner (GP) and as a client by a multidisciplinary team (Clark *et al.* 2004). Their relationships with carers, experts and agencies have apparently been transformed from that envisaged in the initial years of the welfare state as the largely grateful and compliant subjects of state aid. The contemporary service user's need for information and the information needs of the different professionals that may be involved in facilitating and delivering care also become more complex and demanding of local and national data systems.

The *National Service Framework for Older People* (Department of Health 2001a) proposed the introduction of a single assessment process (SAP) for older people from April 2002. This timescale proved somewhat optimistic in view of the obstacles that were encountered. SAP is essentially about information, the gathering of it and the sharing of it between professionals working in health and social care, as well as potentially engaging directly with users. In theory, it should overcome patients'/clients' experiences of giving similar information to any number of people/agencies involved in the delivery of services to them. Frontline professionals such as social workers and community workers who have been trained in the method can undertake the assessments with the expectation that local conditions and established working practices have shaped the form and implementation of SAP. This emphasis on local solutions to the implementation of SAP reflects traditional national/local government divisions that have resulted in different policies, practices and technologies being used in relation to the delivery of services to older people. NHS *Connecting for Health* and the Electronic Social Care Records Implementation Board are involved in an electronic version of SAP (eSAP), which builds on a number of pilot projects that have used laptop computers in meetings between older people and practitioners. This would allow data to be transferred and accessed while the practitioner and client discuss matters over the apocryphal cup of tea. However, a fully functioning electronic service delivery (ESD) system based around eSAP would appear to demand an information system that could be accessed by health and social care practitioners, patients/clients or carers, engage with the NHS Care Records Service (NHS CRS) and act as a resource for management. The intention to provide a 'MyHealthspace' as a 'personalised point of entry to a patient portal through which a patient may access their own health information' suggests that such a level of integration and access may be implemented.

Bodies, sensors and technology

Assistive technology has been defined as 'an umbrella term for any device or system that allows an individual to perform a task that they would otherwise be unable to do or increases the ease and safety with which the task can be performed' (Cowan & Turner-Smith 1999: 81). This highlights the way in which much of the general population makes use of such physically substitutive technology to some degree. However, as one of the authors notes later, this is rather all-embracing and might include eye glasses and contact lenses (Turner-Smith 2000). According to the Audit Commission (2004a: 12), telecare integrates 'electronic assistive technologies' with 'environmental controls', thereby enabling virtual visiting, reminder systems, home security and social alarm systems, thus forming a package that promotes the concept of the 'smart house'. Older people who may benefit from such technology are a heterogeneous group with various degrees of abilities and impairments that do not simply translate into a 'one-fit-all' solution for a particular condition or need. As Dewsbury *et al.* (2004) observe, inclusive and person-centred design and implementation is called for rather than a deficit or 'special needs' approach.

Older bodies living with ill-health may, through SAP and other processes, be categorised as suitable for the use of body monitors and other devices. Such devices include 'WristCare', which monitors the wearer's sleep patterns and movements, and more bodily invasive technologies that render the internal workings of the body into digital data. Devices designed for older people have in common a technology that lifts information out of the body, digitises it and makes it available to often remotely located software and experts. The monitoring of 'vital signs' represents a significant part of the telecare enterprise (Barlow *et al.* 2007). These technologies generate an insistent presence of the medical gaze that may liberate the body from risks and confinements and, at the same time, pathologise and impose new behaviours on the individual. Significantly, a new market has grown up around biosensor devices that make simple measurements of blood pressure and other parameters that can be easily interpreted by the wearer as part of a fitness regime. This self-surveillance of the body by those in pursuit of 'body projects' suggests that older people may also be keen to engage with a similar degree of self-regulation (Shilling 1993).

Mobile devices that have a global positioning system (GPS) capacity represent a modern take on the old location-dependent bell push alarm. What is essentially a mobile phone is marketed by one company as the 'SKeeper' or 'wearable personal safety phone' that allows 'elderly people, children or lone workers to be in close contacts with their relatives or caregivers and get immediate help in case of need from a tele-assistance centre with 24/7 human responses. It enables two-way voice calls and text messages with an advanced alerting system for enhanced personal security. Fully programmable over the air via a user-friendly Web-based interface' (http://www.medinfonews.com/ar/6y.htm). The European MobilAlarm project integrates GPS, mobile telephony and body-worn sensor devices with service centres and geographical localisation and alerting software to provide a Europe-wide mobile alarm and tele-assistance service (http://www.mobilalarm-eu.org). These and other projects use existing technologies such as the mobile phone and other network systems to create services dedicated to older people and those with chronic conditions in ways that potentially allow them mobility and an escape from the home that they had not previously enjoyed. Such technologies are not without ethical and other problems. For example, people with dementia, who may wander without knowing where they are, can be subject to surveillance through a location-sensitive device such as a radio frequency identity (RFID) tag that promises to enhance their safety and independence. Equally, it can be argued that such strategies infantilise the user and pathologise behaviours that are not predicable and routine, thus narrowing their scope for 'normal' modes of social interaction and movement.

Home is where the technology is

In the 1980s, there was much hype around the idea of the 'telecottage' that promised to help regenerate rural areas and transform mundane working lives by making it possible to work at a distance. However, smart homes might be capable of far more:

> They walked down the hall of their soundproofed Happylife Home, which had cost them thirty thousand dollars installed, this house which clothed and fed and rocked them to sleep and played and sang and was good to them. Their approach sensitized a switch somewhere and the nursery light flicked on when they came within ten feet of it. Similarly, behind them, in the halls, lights went on and off as they left them behind, with a soft automaticity.
>
> Bradbury (1995: 56)

Ray Bradbury's short science fiction story neatly captures the seductive and subversive nature of the technologically rich home. Indeed, the 'Happylife Home' has resonances with the technology that it is claimed is used by the founder of Microsoft in his home:

> Visitors to Bill Gates House are surveyed and given a microchip upon entrance. This small chip sends signals throughout the house, and a given room's temperature and other conditions will change according to preset user preferences.
>
> http://labnol.blogspot.com/2005/05/inside-bill-gates-home.html

However, these homes were designed to enhance and extend bodies that did not suffer from any loss of health or capacity. A number of demonstrator smart homes have been constructed in Edinburgh, York and Gloucester to show the potential of technology for different user groups. As Hanson, Osipovič and Percival (Chapter 7) argue, much work needs to be done in order to understand how older people use and interact with such technology. Technological interventions in the homes occupied by ageing or ill bodies have tended to restore previous bodily capacities or to contribute to the ability of an individual to remain independent by moving the site of body monitoring from the clinic to the home. Reductionist definitions of disability that focus upon ambulatory and/or mobility issues have too often shaped technology in the home (Imrie 2003). Indeed, the degree to which such initiatives are effective in terms of organisational costs is largely unclear (Lancet 1995; Roine *et al.* 2001). The cost to the occupiers of such smart homes may be their sense of privacy as surveillance systems, and especially those that include video devices, stream data to unknown software and human watchers (see Chapter 7). While there appear to be ever increasing amounts of digital information available, it is less clear whether the software and human recipients of the data are capable of making meaningful and nuanced observations and decision based on it. Percival, Hanson and Osipovič (Chapter 4) highlight the need for proper training and support for staff if such innovations are to be implemented effectively.

One of the earliest telecare systems in the UK was an integrated alarm system built into a 1948 sheltered housing scheme in Devon that sounded a bell in the warden's accommodation (Parry & Thompson 1993). Fisk (1989) argues that this association with housing led to a 'property rather than person-based perspective' that resonates across the various shifts in the organisation of housing, social services and health care in the UK. Since then, technology has move on apace and witnessed the revolution led by the microchip so that the simple bell push has evolved into integrated telecare systems. The electro-mechanical devices of what has been seen as the first generation of telecare systems have been superseded by new 'intelligent' systems. Acting through sensors, the body and the home can be monitored so that an alarm is issued independently of any conscious effort on the part of the older person. The third generation of technologies includes 'lifestyle monitoring' such as devices that monitor when a fridge is used as well as recognising the possibilities that fast Internet connectivity can provide for older people (Doughty *et al*. 1996; Chapters 6 and 9). The potential of the Internet was highlighted in the Department of Trade and Industry (DTI) expectations for health care in 2020 when ' ... the first point of contact with health care will be through a "virtual" cyber-physician (CP). Accessed through a TV screen, the CP will replace other forms of triage such as the telephone and give access to infor-mation about other professionals, hospitals and other aspects of health care' (Department of Trade and Industry 2000: 18). There is a danger in such expeditions into futurology as there is a temptation to extrapolate social and policy developments from assumptions about technological change.

The apparent virtualisation of care draws attention the to role of the Inter-net. Those over 55 years of age remain under-represented among Internet users in the UK (Dutton & Helsper 2007). For those for whom digital technology did not form part of their working lives, the computer may be unfamiliar, and there is a need for training and support of a kind provided by various 'silver surfers' and other schemes (Pilling *et al*. 2004). However, when access is uti-lised to make contact with family and friends as well as working on hobbies, this has encouraged a move to use the Internet for as much as seven hours a day according to one survey undertaken for a financial services group (AXA 2007). Featherstone (1995) suggests that 'technological modes of interchange' can transcend bodily limitations to 'open up new possibilities for intimacy and self-expression' (ibid.: 612). Indeed, some research has claimed that older people who are Internet users have a greater sense of psychological well-being than non-users and hence a sense of empowerment (Chen & Persons 2002; Chapter 9). Access to the Internet may bring many benefits, but the virtual is no substitute for embodied social interaction. The majority of Internet services are primarily aimed at those who can read English and, despite the availability of, for example, online retail services, the attendant websites are designed around assumptions about 'normal' users and fail to cater to the needs of minority groups (Barlow & Breeze 2005). Online shopping is convenient but, for many people, the act of shopping (even in a supermarket) is about social contact that requires a move from the home. Equally, while the virtual consultation with practitioners suggested by the DTI may be efficient in terms of their time, it may conversely lead to feelings of isolation and have implications for individuals' sense of well-being (see Chapter 8). The people who are the subject of this book are all too aware of the visceral, physical body so that mediated interactions that leave the body behind may prove to be attractive. However, they may also choose to keep their bodies, if not identities, as part of their online interaction. There may be advantages here as shared experiences can help generate a sense of community and promote mutual support (Burrows *et al.* 2000; Hardey 2004; Seymore & Lupton 2004). Such digital spaces should be seen as running alongside rather than displacing material sociability. Telephone-based support services such as that discussed by Reed (Chapter 9), which allow 'conferencing' among users, may perform similar functions. Such meditative technologies can open up new opportunities and offer new forms of sociability, but this does not mean that older people can be assumed to be happily and safely confined to a real version of a 'Happylife Home' in a parody of the dystopian visions of the never offline computer gamer.

The chapters of this book in context

A virtue of an edited book is that it can bring together a variety of perspectives informed by a range of studies and disciplines. The book falls into three sections. The first section deals with policy and the integration of services. Following this introduction, the initial chapter by Rob Wilson and Sue Baines draws attention to the rationale behind the integration of care for older people and uses empirical studies to highlight the pitfalls and potential benefits. Based on a study of older people, the following chapters examine how the integration and informatisation of services have been implemented. Leigh Keeble, Brian Loader and Michael Hardey reveal how the escalating number of government changes to welfare delivery and related policy initiatives may hinder the process of informatisation. The second section explores the role of older people in shaping the technologies that might be available to them. It opens with John Percival, Julienne Hanson and Dorota Osipovič's report on research that examined users' beliefs about telehealth technologies. This suggests that older people may be keen to make use of such technology provided practitioners support them. The latter are clear about the implications this demand has for their training and resource need. Andrew Webster's chapter takes a more theoretical approach to informatisation and the way it gives users new responsibilities. He also situates health technologies within the broader literature about information and communication technologies (ICTs) and health policy in relation to the reconfiguration of the role of the patient. The last chapter in this section gives John Powell an opportunity to examine how Internet support groups contribute to the lives of carers of people with dementia. Drawing on a number of studies, he argues that there is a lack of evidence that virtual support groups can address the needs of carers. In particular, the danger of inflating the potential of technology, previously highlighted by Andrew Webster, is reflected here in a critique of the assumption that ICTs are empowering. The final section focuses on the importance of the role of design and the integration of users into all levels of implementation. Julienne Hanson, Dorota Osipovič and John Percival look at a number of pilot projects that have implemented telecare devices in homes to establish lifestyle monitoring. They argue that such levels of monitoring place considerable demands on the interpretation of the consequent data that cannot simply be regarded as a digital flow from one aspect of an individual's routine but are rather embedded in the messy reality of everyday life. In the subsequent chapter, Darren Reed undertakes an exploration of telephone support services. Drawing on a 'performative turn' approach, he, like Julienne Hanson, Dorota Osipovič and John Percival, highlights the need for the telecare support services to be seen and assessed in the context of the users' mundane lives and practices. In the final chapter, Sally McMillan, Elizabeth Johnson Avery and Wendy Macias draw on the experiences of older people in the United States to argue that mediated communication can provide a sense of empowerment and belonging.

Making connections in context

As the chapters of this book argue, the provision of technologies for older people is evidently both complex and open to various levels of implementation and interpretation. Present and future informatisational assistive systems and technologies are shaped by past configurations and policies. Furthermore, there is a tendency for work within the various 'tele' and 'informational' categories to become the focus within particular specialisms or areas of practice. In an attempt to understand the forces at work here and place in context the various issues raised in the chapters in this book, a typology has been developed. It should be treated as an ideal type with the usual caveats, but the typology is based on an examination of the extant evidence at both policy and empirical level. As we have seen, the integration of services in both the material sense (e.g. interagency teams) and the technological sense (e.g. NHS CRS 'spine') is a key policy driver and has resulted in more or less successful implementation at both local and national level. However, as Wilson (Chapter 2) argues, the legacy of previous policies and systems has an influence on new technologies and initiatives. This is mapped onto the typology at a high and a low level on the vertical axis, with high representing a fully integrated service and low the opposite case. The user (whatever the label used) is now placed centrally at both policy and practice level. Engagement relates to the way in which users are incorporated within the practices that arise from the delivery of services and is mapped on a low/high continuum on the horizontal axis. This typology generates four ideal type models, which are outlined in Table 1.1. The scope and complexity of informational systems varies across the models. Each model is discussed with the implications for informatisation and the practitioner/user relationship highlighted.

Table 1.1 A typology of informatisation

	User engagement low	User engagement high
Integration low	1. Past practice	2. Pilot studies
Integration high	3. Emergent practice	4. Future prospects

1 Past practice

The model labelled 'past practice' represents the organisational structure(s) and practices in health and social care that grew out of the development of the welfare state. It represents a time when the delivery of health and social services was characterised by vertical control and professional differentiation (for example between health practitioners and social workers). Evolving divisions between national and local services became a central concern of the modernising agenda of the 1980s and a driver for much consequent change. Past practices have left a legacy of often incompatible technologies and data (see Chapter 2). Subject to what has been described as the 'technology push', telecare was often implemented in a technological determinist way that failed to take account of nuanced human action and anxieties (Moran 1993). Lack of consistent planning at local and national level in relation to telecare provided little incentive for commercial interests to develop new devices aimed at an uncertain market (Doughty & Williams 2001). Moreover, the relatively slow rate of development in the UK of good-quality cable networks acted as a brake on innovations that required reliable and inexpensive digital connectivity (Pragnell *et al.* 2000). Past practice also highlights what is now considered to be a 'heritage problem', whereby parts of the health and welfare system, at both national and local level, have independent IT systems with a limited ability to exchange information digitally. The user is seen largely as an information provider to experts who are trusted and expected to make important decisions about their clients' care. The Parsonian (1951) model of expert/user relationships is largely intact and valued by practitioners, who can exercise their professional judgement and intuition, and by users who have faith in professionals and are happy to comply with their recommendations. The status and divisions of the various practitioners that may be involved in assessing and delivering care remain important. Face-to-face contact with practitioners is central to the assessment and delivery of care and reinforced by the various divides including those between housing, general practice and nursing services. Local solutions to health and care delivery reflect budgetary and other divisions at local and national level.

2 Pilot studies

In the course of the informatisation of social and health care, there have been any number of pilot projects and trials that have built systems and technologies in order to test or point to possible routes to implementation, e.g. 'At

Home and in Touch', Durham County Council; 'The Columbia Project', 'Framework for Multi-agency Environments' (FRAME) pilots (see Chapters 2 and 8). Many of these projects engage in careful user modelling, which may drive innovations forward. Informatisation pilots broadly presuppose the existence of something like eSAP supported by a national information system. The role of practitioners is largely seen as delivering therapy and negotiating care in an established fashion. Some pilot studies have an image of the users at the centre of an information system where health and social care is one possible area of interest among other options that include email, shopping and travel. In this model, IT is seen as formative to consumer life and, as such, it holds a vision of a common interface through which all e-services can be easily accessed. It is possible to envisage a system that may be voice controlled and includes data from any telecare technologies so that the older person is in the centre of a data stream that is dedicated to their needs and more or less at their direction. Valuable data may be obtained from these pilots, but many nonetheless remain on the fringe of mainstream service provision as a consequence of their need for high integration to be fully implemented.

3 Emergent practice

This model assumes that informatisation remains fractured and underlying delivery structures are divided territorially and in other ways. It is emergent because it reflects the current situation across England and Wales. There is an emerging national integrated IT system across health and social services with more or less integrated databases (Department of Health 2007). SAP is a key portal for users to negotiate their needs, but they are more or less reliant on the skills and knowledge of practitioners to 'manage' the welfare on their behalf. Older people are excluded from system design aspects, and limited if any use has been made of user modelling within the various IT systems. The Warner review notes that integration of telecare has implications for staff and practitioner roles at all levels (King's Fund 2006). However, the general exclusion of frontline staff from various implementation processes has resulted in resistance from practitioners. The development of integrated teams remains at an early stage in some areas, while in others there are fully functional groups (see Chapter 3). A traditional expert-down model of design and implementation has been seen as necessary to deal with the complexity of pre-existing databases and the technical demands made of the system. In this model, IT is essentially a managerial tool so that various manifestations of it are designed around the requirements of, for example, case management, target setting and resource allocation. It also enables local and national elements of the health and social care structure to 'go their own way' and make arrangements for their own IT and care delivery systems, which, while tailored to their needs, are incompatible with systems used elsewhere. This has proved problematic, especially among GP practices and in relation to such systems as *Choose and Book*.

Local policies and practices remain important in shaping telecare opportunities and have given rise to a range of innovative pilots and trials noted previously. Policy changes symbolised by direct payments and manifest in the SAP provide new opportunities for users to have a potentially central role in negotiating their needs. A broad shift in the recognition of users as consumers of services is challenging the image of older people as 'frail'. Moreover, recognition of the 'grey pound' by the commercial sector is increasing the marketisation of technologies in this market where people have choices that may lead to a greater sense of control and independence (Fisk 2003). However, many users remain as the more or less unwired 'customers' in a mixed economy of care that is negotiated for them by practitioners who can develop expertise in negotiating different policies, practices and priorities. In effect, it represents a limited informatisation of older people who become subject to data collection rather than having a reflexive engagement with the system(s).

4 Future prospects

This represents the fulfilment of the long established policy vision of integrated services and 'joined up' government, at both local and national level, that is successful in providing reliable information at the point of use. Informed by the possibilities manifest in various pilot projects, this model also embraces telecare as integral where necessary to information systems. The model is driven by the implementation of policies that were supported by previous research and careful planning. Design and implementation decisions were made centrally with clear criteria provided so that local areas could amend the systems to meet local conditions. Care is delivered seamlessly based on user needs that are established by ongoing negotiation between a key practitioner and the user which is mediated through eSAP. This negotiation is more or less virtual in that initial assessments may be conducted face to face with the aid of a dedicated laptop or other mobile devices that can interact with other data stored remotely and, where appropriate, arrange services and resources. Subsequent changes may be made directly through the information system, which can include the ability for consultations to take place online. Older people, carers, practitioners and others involved in delivering care to any individual have access to one common interface where they can contribute information, make and track decisions and so forth. This interface and some of the data policies and practices that underlie it have emerged from a careful process of user modelling and various pilot studies to ensure that older people and others can easily access it. In addition, care has been taken to ensure that the design is inclusive and so can make use of minority languages, levels of disability and so forth. It is likely that future generations of older people will be increasingly familiar with technology and may adopt a more consumerist attitude to public services than the generation who experienced life before the development of the NHS. Indeed, the policy vision may incorporate a broader model in which data are shared across state agencies unconstrained by privacy legislation and practice. It is possible to see this model produce an image of a global user-centred interface to all state, commercial and other services that would draw on collective user-centred activities evident in current manifestations of Web 2.0. For example, users could rate/review services, products or practitioners in a similar fashion to customers of Amazon reviewing the purchases they have made or leaving recommendations for others.

Data, like care, are seamlessly, securely and dynamically shared among all those involved with the delivery of service to a particular individual. This would apparently promote efficiency and end the duplication of data input to offer a further degree of seamless government service to individual citizens who can be defined by their identity card. Moreover, there is scope for data to transcend national boundaries, especially within the European Union (EU), so that health care information becomes exchangeable. However, the possibilities of surveillance increase significantly, and questions about who owns data about an individual, some of which is user generated, must be considered. The Audit Commission (2004a) suggests that telecare technologies may reduce reliance on human agency and a fully integrated information/sensor system may meet users' needs before they themselves may be aware of them. However, all utopias have a dark side, and users may be recast as subjects of 'dataveillence' so that, while their needs might be met, their choices are prescribed as they are socially sorted to provide the optimal delivery of care (Lyon 2003). This raises the question of how far the mediation of services should go in addressing the needs of users? It is not difficult to envisage a system that, while empowering users through their computer, may actually reduce their face-to-face contact with others (especially in view of the financial pressures on day care centres and so forth), discourage mobility and fitness and generally adversely affect well-being. Indeed, while it is generally held that telecare resources are liberating in the sense that they 'fix' bodily inadequacies combined with other technologies (some of which are glimpsed in the smart home), they may also evolve to discipline bodies. Video and other forms of surveillance or lifestyle monitoring will develop further and may disappear within technologies (e.g. alarm systems, the computer, etc.), renewing the need to understand the boundaries around public and private information and spaces. Whether the cost of such systems will be seen as offering the state or individuals 'value for money' is questionable. Some form of digital inequality will persist, and it is possible that those who demand face-to-face service delivery will receive a residual service as traditional methods are marginalised in the face of high costs and increased reliance on an integrated and mediated health and social care system. Finally, a fully integrated or shared information system across state agencies may create a new category of 'system outcasts', who may be victims of data errors or found not to be entitled to citizenship rights and therefore subject to expulsion or other sanctions.

Part I

Towards integrated service provision?

2 Are there limits to the integration of care for older people?

Rob Wilson and Sue Baines

Introduction

Information and communications technologies (ICTs) in the domain of health are seen by national governments, including the UK, as key to the modernising of health and social care. IT solutions are now being put in place across the country and are expected to deliver a diverse set of joining-up agendas across medicine and social care, including prevention strategies, chronic disease management and the facilitation of active participation of patients and enabling personalisation of care. Against a background of the overarching policy requirement of service integration, this chapter will explore and reflect upon the recent history of the care of older people in England. It will do this through the lens of the single assessment process (SAP). SAP is intended to ensure joined-up care for older people by supporting interorganisational and interprofessional information sharing. SAP systems across England, however, are not all the same. On the contrary, they have been begun from different starting points and been implemented locally with different technologies, organisational practices and governance structures, adding up to a series of local 'organisational aquariums' where at any point the full range of behaviours between their organisational inhabitants are observable. We will draw upon examples of some of this diverse SAP experience to challenge the idea that the current approaches to service integration (generally point to point between statutory organisations) represent a sustainable scalable solution to the problem of sharing information and knowledge in public sector domains.

Why integrate care for older people?

People aged 65 and over make up around 16 per cent of the UK population, but this group accounts for more than two-fifths (43 per cent) of the total budget of the National Health Service and nearly three-fifths (58 per cent) of local authority social services' budgets (Philip 2007). Rapidly increasing demand from older people for services is one of the complex social problems (sometimes called 'wicked' problems) that demand co-coordinated activities across organisational boundaries or 'holistic' government (6 *et al.* 2002; Ling 2002).

For older adults, joining-up problems and their solutions in England are usually framed around the half-century-old split between health and social care. Responsibility for older adults was divided between the National Health Service (NHS) and local authorities at the inception of the welfare state. This division resulted in interminable struggles between separate institutions to delineate their respective responsibilities (Lewis 2001; Reed *et al.* 2005). Reforms of the 1980s and 1990s that included the introduction of contracting and quasi-markets contributed to the further sharpening of organisational and service boundaries. Legacies of that history still persist, although many older people's needs exist on the borders of both 'health' and 'care', and older people themselves are unlikely to define their needs as either 'health' or 'care' (Lymbery 2006). Since the turn of the century, joining up of health and care services for older people has been emphasised in a series of policy documents, including *Information for Health* (Department of Health 1998), *Information for Social Care* (Department of Health 2001b) and *Delivering 21st Century IT Support for the NHS* (Department of Health 2002b). The importance of ICTs to enable joining up across the health/social care divide has been highlighted in the *Vision for Adult Social Care* (Department of Health 2005b), the Health Select Committee Report of 2005. The White Paper, *Our Health, Our Care, Our Say* (Department of Health 2006) presents a vision of care for adults that is person centred, seamless and will make better use of technology.

At the same time as it demands joined-up, 'person-centred' services, central government is putting in place mechanisms to harness the contributions of a much more diverse range of partner organisations to tackle social and health inequalities (Secretary of State 2006). The *Cross Cutting Review* (HM Treasury 2002) called upon all government departments to work more effectively with the voluntary and community sector. *Our Health, Our Care, Our Say* (Department of Health 2006) highlighted third sector organisations (including social enterprises) as an important means of raising the quality of services. The following year *World Class Commissioning* (Department of Health 2007b) called for more new 'independent' providers from the third and private sectors in the health care market to stimulate innovation, drive up standards and respond to patients' needs. Visions for the future encompass an increasingly diverse array of providers and partnership arrangements; new vehicles for delivery feature joint ventures with the private and voluntary sectors, community partnerships for health and well-being, local businesses and community self-help groups (Dawson *et al.* 2007).

Recent policies to overcome the historic health/social care divide have been described as 'vertical' integration (Reed *et al.* 2005) or 'deep' integration (Glasby 2007). Examples of this type of integration are pooled funding arrangements and the restructuring of different types of care (e.g. acute and long term) under one administrative umbrella. Glasby (2007) argues that deep integration across the health/social care divide in adult services contrasts with broader and shallower (also described by Reed *et al.* 2005 as 'horizontal') forms of integration that have become typical in children's services. Yet older people's lives are affected by services beyond the domains of health and social care, for example housing, transport, leisure and a plethora of so-called 'low level' interventions typically offered by the voluntary and community sector. In short, in older people's services, as in those for children and young people, there are increasingly complex sets of relationships and responsibilities with partners and service providers.

'Integration', nevertheless, remains a persistent discourse in the most recent policy documents, for example: 'PCTs and local authorities are expected to develop *integrated* approaches to achieve specific outcomes for their local populations, including universal information, advice and advocacy' (DH/ADASS/LGA/NHS 2007). A view from a largely clinical perspective reinforces the two-dimensional perspective which layers the care of older people into 'rings' of an increasingly specialised service provision. Such 'onion' models (e.g. Figure 2.1) are common in health and social care policy and strategy documents and explicitly reflect the aim of models of service integration and person-centred care.

It remains questionable whether the tools and technologies currently in use support the drive towards diversity in service provision and are flexible enough to respond to coordination, collaboration and networking demands between the statutory and non-statutory agencies and individual professionals, carers and patients. Drawing on the recent experience of SAP, we illustrate our concern that current technical configurations tend to be envisaged for 'deep–vertical' integrations that fail to respond to the increasingly diverse service environment. Limits to the sustainability and scalability of such integration are among the hardest lessons from SAP.

Single assessment process – a deep integration approach?

This section will describe and analyse the recent history of the SAP. After an overview of the policies and expectations that underpinned the principles of SAP, we focus upon four local projects tasked with creating a working SAP

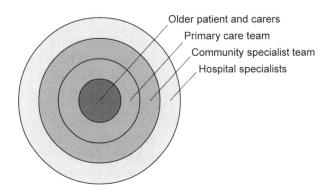

Older patient and carers
Primary care team
Community specialist team
Hospital specialists

Figure 2.1 Rings of change partnership model (from Philip 2007)

approach to the care integration problem. These projects were initiated and governed differently, but all concentrated on integration between statutory agencies, in other words conforming to the 'deep' or 'vertical' approach described above. The orthodoxy of integration is critiqued in the context of the reality of emerging networks of multiagency service delivery and coordination. This critique directly challenges the idea that integration is a sustainable, scalable solution to the problem of coordination and personalisation of the care and welfare services for older people where interorganisational and cross-sector information sharing is required.

SAPs are intended to provide a common approach to sharing information, thereby improving coordination, referral and discharge between the different parts of the statutory care network. In England, for older people, a SAP was initially mooted in the National Health Service Plan at the turn of the century and was introduced in full through the third National Service Framework (NSF), which aimed to directly improve the care of older people (National Service Framework for Older People 2001). Raising standards of care was at the heart of the NSF for Older People, and one of the central themes of the new policy direction was to deliver personalised commissioning and care services. The NSF sets out national standards and service models of care across health and social services for all older people whether in domiciliary, residential or health care contexts. The standards outlined in 2001 covered a range of service issues including (National Service Framework for Older People 2001):

- Standard one: rooting out age discrimination
- Standard two: person-centred care
- Standard three: intermediate care
- Standard four: general hospital care
- Standard five: stroke
- Standard six: falls
- Standard seven: mental health in older people
- Standard eight: the promotion of health and active life in older age.

One of the major arguments held up in favour of moving to a SAP at the time of the NSF (under Standard 2) was clinical research evidence for the success of structured assessment approaches to deliver strong long-term management and effective support for survival and function in older persons (Stuck *et al.* 1993). Following the publication of the NSF, the implementation of SAP began in earnest as a process tool for delivering the emerging 'whole systems' agenda (see Change Agent Team, DH 2004). SAPs were developed and deployed as a set of paper-based or computer-based forms that structure the practitioner assessment processes. They used a range of formal structured assessment process tools, based on forms including combinations of tick boxes, validated assessment scores and some free text. The forms could be locally developed but in the main were off-the-shelf products, developed and validated in a variety of contexts. We now introduce projects from two contrasting work programmes that implemented SAP at the local level in England. One of these programmes was led by local government social services and the other by the NHS. We consider some of the contrasts and commonalities between them before proposing lessons for the integration agenda from their successes and setbacks. The evidence upon which we draw is based upon our close involvement with both programmes.

The responsibility for the delivery of SAP was given initially by central government to local authority Directors of Social Services, partially in the context of media interest in the problem of 'bed blocking' – where patients could not be discharged from hospital into the community until an assessment had been completed. Local authorities in England with social service responsibilities were set a target for the implementation of a single assessment system (either paper or computer based) of April 2004. During this period, the central government department responsible for local government (then the Office of the Deputy Prime Minister – ODPM; now the Department for Communities and Local Government – DCLG) began a programme of projects for supporting the delivery of local e-government in line with the context of a wider national drive for e-enabling services. One of the projects addressed the requirements of the 'joining-up' agenda across a selection of social care contexts. This was known as FAME (Framework for Multi-agency Environments). In common with the rest of the local e-government programme, FAME was expected to demonstrate the ability of ICT to support improvements in effectiveness and efficiency in specific service instances in local government areas, with the ultimate aim of 'shrink-wrapping' products and lessons learned to make 'best practice' transferable to other similar service contexts. The first local SAP projects considered here were led by local authorities under the auspices of FAME. Both authors were part of a team from Newcastle University's Centre for Social and Business Informatics (SBI) which was a partner in the FAME project. One of SBI's roles in FAME was evaluation of the local projects (for more details, see Baines *et al.* 2004). Data from the FAME evaluation used in this chapter are: Transcripts of meetings with project managers, project officers and other key individuals, e.g. project 'champions' (based on four visits over the life of the project to each of two local SAP sites); field notes on observations of events, workshops and project meetings; and documents, e.g. board minutes and local reports to the national project.

During its first phase, the FAME project (April 2003–October 2004) developed and deployed information systems at a local authority level. Six local pilot projects (known within the FAME project as 'strands') were each led by an English local authority in partnership with other service providers. Each 'strand' aimed to produce a working 'whole system' (including a technical system) for the exchange and management of client/patient information across agency and professional boundaries in a specific policy priority service context (e.g. for mental health or older people) within the local authority area. Two IT suppliers worked with FAME as 'technology partners'. FAME faced delays mainly because the technical interoperatability of service-level applications proved more intractable than anticipated. For example, the supplier of social care systems to several participating local authorities announced that their new product to enable the technology partners to extract data would become available in autumn 2003. By spring 2004, there was still no extract routine to get data out of existing record systems. Relationships between this supplier and the FAME project became increasingly fraught. The technology partners were frustrated by the impasse and complained bitterly that local authority partners failed to progress the issue because they were beholden to their main suppliers. Only two of the six strands achieved the promised technical implementation on schedule (i.e. by May 2004). All of them delivered a set of non-technical products including an information sharing protocol (a document describing in legal terms the information to be shared by all the participating organisations), a log of lessons learned and a business case. (These products are available through the project website archive at http://www.fame-uk.org.)

One of the two FAME strands that was successful in implementing the ICT system component, more or less on schedule, produced an electronic SAP for older adults. This strand involved two separate (but cooperating) sites, one in the north of England and one in the south. In each site, the project teams managed to maintain the partnership across health and social care, but this was a formidable and time-consuming task, always precarious and contingent upon the energy and commitment of a few individuals (Gannon-Leary *et al.* 2006; Wilson *et al.* 2007). The difficulty of working across the health/social care divide is well documented, and the challenges in this respect were foreseen and, for the most part, successfully mitigated by project planning and hard work. There were, however, unforeseen tensions that raised more difficult questions about the nature and limits of ICT-enabled integration in older people's services.

Referrals to the central duty team (social services) were usually from third parties – such as neighbours or family – who cannot give consent to sharing personal information about individuals with others. The difficulty was overcome with a workaround by referring the case within the local authority to the social services or occupational therapy service, which would later need to seek consent from the user to share information with other agencies. The problem is important because it illustrates how boundaries around agencies can be defined and managed in complex multiagency environments and how the contributions of families and informal carers can be recognised.

One of the partners in the northern SAP site was a service provider from the voluntary sector. (The southern site had only statutory partners.) There was already a local information sharing protocol (ISP), which the project adopted as a convenient short cut. It transpired after most of the partners thought the ISP was in place that it did not take account of the voluntary sector and had to be hastily revised to do so, at some cost to progressing the project.

The most dramatic setback was when general practitioners (GPs) in the northern FAME SAP site had to be disconnected from the system soon after it went live. These GPs were furious when they discovered that they could see the names of each other's patients. GPs thought it was obvious that this integration of patient information would be unacceptable (they believed that it contradicted their terms of service). Nobody else in the project, including the technology partner, was aware of the issue until it became a crisis that delayed the project.

All the FAME strands including the SAP sites had the objective of producing a multiagency, single-service, single-locality implementation. From the setbacks and challenges they faced, there are two specific warnings for future attempts to implement service integration enabled by ICT:

- 'Overintegration' of data resulted in resistance from practitioners (when decontextualised information about service users could be viewed by other practitioners)
- The limitations of local solutions that failed to accommodate the roles of non-statutory participants (voluntary sector organisations and neighbours, carers and friends of service users).

Following on in late 2003, the Connecting for Health (CfH) National Programme for IT (NPfIT) was initiated. The first phase of the programme activity culminated in the issuing of an 'output-based specification' (OBS) document, which included a specification for a computer-based SAP. Subsequent phases of NPfIT led to contracts being let for core parts of the NPfIT functionality (e.g. the national summary record or 'spine') or for one of five regional local services providers (LSPs) who contracted to deliver a range of organisational (e.g. for hospitals) or care community-level applications (e.g. SAP). Two of the five regional clusters were contracted to deliver SAP systems to local care communities in their initial implementation phase. The examples discussed here are from two locality implementations from one of these regional clusters (http://www.cfh.nhs.uk).

The e-SAP team (whose responsibility was to take forward the concept of SAP as a national service) consulted Newcastle University researchers including one of the authors (Wilson) on the strength of their work on the FAME project. The observations and data on local issues cited in this section are based on documents and relationships within one region (the north-east of England) and on participation in local events including practitioner/manager conferences and a lessons learned review (http://www.cpa.org.uk/sap/sap_about.html; http://www.cfh.nhs.uk).

The first locality we consider was one of the earliest of the CfH-led SAP implementations. It was carried out in 2004 and was dogged by a number of difficulties before the implementation process started, including a high level of confidence on the part of health service leaders, some existing poor relationships with and between technology system suppliers (both within and outside the NPfIT cluster LSP contract) and a lack of engagement and communication between the parties about existing implementations and future arrangements for SAP. This last point led to animated discussions between local government, health service managers, cluster representatives and LSPs about the planning, local delivery and benefits realisation activity.

The second CfH SAP locality was one of the more successful initial implementations of SAP in the regional CfH cluster. The locality has a history of partnership working between social services and health. In the case of older people, the organisations involved had, as an initial priority, established joint momentum at the director, management and practitioner level. Agreements were reached early on about the governance structure of the local SAP project (the emphasis being on health improvement for older people), which appears to have laid the foundation for work towards the development with the initial Department of Health (DH) target of April 2004. The partnership had put considerable effort and resources (including engagement of practitioners, governance arrangements and local facilitation work) into producing a locality-specific draft paper-based system which, after a relatively short period of use (which demonstrated the problem of implementing distributed paper-based systems), was upgraded to one of the accredited tools in a computer-based system on offer from CfH. Since the initially successful implementation, the governance structures of the local health trust have changed to be merged with two other local trusts. The long-term sustainability of the integration is potentially in question as the forces that led to the integration being achieved initially are likely to be dissipated as time goes on.

The objective of the FAME SAP and CfH SAP projects was to deliver working electronic single assessment tools designed to improve the way older people are jointly assessed for their health and social care needs. Embedded within the electronic tool was one of a small number of assessment instruments accredited by the DH which could also be used in paper form. Based on a similar technical approach and assessment tools, the SAP applications aimed to support practitioners across participating statutory agencies to improve the care of older people. However, the structure of the implementations in between the projects discussed above was quite different in terms of the governance of the technical activity. The governance of the CfH applications was located on the health care structures at the CfH regional cluster level and subregional level (in Strategic Health Authorities – SHAs), rather than at local authority/primary care trust (locality) level in the FAME project SAPs.

Various delays led to patchy results within implementation sites with, for example, training on the system being conducted several weeks before the technical system went live. A number of further contextual issues also confounded the implementation process in the locality including: a lack of coherent leadership due to a number of ongoing organisational changes; mixed success in historical local attempts to integrate between health and social care organisations; high priority for innovations in the children's services domain, which stretched scarce resources in the local government organisations involved.

Once initiated, all the case studies' implementation processes ran into technical delays (including the technical interoperability of service-level applications, e.g. social work systems). The problem across the cases was basically conceived as a lack of data integration between the new SAP application and the existing record systems. The solution to the problem is widely framed as a need for system integration within and between public sector organisations (and indeed more widely). In the case of SAP, this is typically in the background of a longer term reliance on IT to support the handling of information in an ever wider range of institutional or directorate business processes (including supporting the production of management information for central government, supporting inspection and automating archiving). Such systems often run in parallel to paper or *ad hoc* email-based practices. It is this proliferation of systems that gives rise to the basic integration problem. A second important trend has been the long-established rise in computer-based information systems and the decline in paper-based information systems in a number of core systems areas (administrative systems, record systems, etc.). In many of these areas, a relatively small number of specialist vendors (often led by ex-professionals from the particular domain) tend to dominate in a context where the market has become saturated with long-established 'shrink-wrapped' application product sets often with inherent legacy problems (for instance, see Sugden *et al.* 2008). Within these diverse contexts (e.g. primary care, social services and the voluntary sector), record-keeping practices and information use vary widely within and across the agencies involved, for instance in the context of health records.

In particular, GP records make use of extensive coding and tend to be primarily used by other GPs/health care staff within a practice, whereas social service records tend to comprise significant detail about clients and their social context in relatively unstructured narrative form, which supports a wider set of audiences (including other social workers, other professionals in case meetings, social service inspectors and the clients themselves). This is also partly reflected in the level of investment in information systems. For instance, in this context, social service systems have often received 'Cinderella' levels of funding compared with the 'ugly sisters' of e-health and e-government.

Within the case studies, it became clear that the sheer number and diversity of partners in some deployments of multiagency working meant that no single vendor could legitimately provide the niche functionality and specialised support required, and so a range of common integration problems has emerged between the offerings of this restricted set of system vendors with overlapping business models. Attempts by new vendors or products to enter the space between organisation/service-specific system applications are often beset with 'turf wars' and heavily disputed 'technical integration costs' between the organisations and suppliers' IT sections.

Overall, evidence from these contrasting SAP implementations demonstrates that the challenges of successful 'deep' integration of care require approaches that take in diverse characteristics including technical integration, shared governance, established trust between partners, enthusiasm and energy of committed individuals, staff training and sustained commitment at a strategic level.

The experience of these SAP project case studies which attempted to create 'deep–vertical' integrations, on the whole between the statutory agencies (NHS organisations and local government social service departments) reaffirms the evidence that, despite the political, legislative and strategic pressure to create 'tightly coupled' (Wieck 2001) interprofessional partnership working, the resulting integrations tend to be limited, unstable and contingent on local circumstances. In fact, in at least one instance, we observed that 'over-integration' had taken place in the context of patient information being shared inappropriately between GPs.

Forming and maintaining partnerships are terribly familiar challenges in multiagency working, which were anticipated as risks within the projects and addressed, at least in part, by mitigating action by project managers and others during the main periods of activity. The development process of the SAP pilots also highlighted a number of other issues familiar in the literature in this area, which shows that improving the integration of care is not uniformly successful in improving practice. First, the literature suggests that the integration of care has been overly focused on the organisational aspects of integration at the expense of practice/interprofessional working elements (e.g. Challis *et al.* 2006; van Wijngaarden *et al.* 2006), that there is only ambiguous evidence of the efficiency, effectiveness and overall success rate of attempts at integration (e.g. Evers *et al.* 2001; Wan *et al.* 2001; Glasby 2004) and that the ongoing challenges of reshaping organisational, partnership working, governance and professional cultures remain largely unchanged despite significant emphasis in some areas (Worth 2001; Hudson 2002; Dickinson 2006).

Many of these issues have been reiterated repeatedly in the policy and academic literature, most recently in the Commission for Social Care Inspection's annual report to parliament, *The State of Social Care in England 2006–7*, where evidence is reported of diverse practice in the interpretation of criteria by local practitioners making assessments of older people (Commission for Social Care Inspection 2008).

Is integration really the *only* answer to the question of improving service coordination?

ICT-based information systems have proliferated in NHS and local government organisations, particularly in recent years. This proliferation of systems, however, has not taken place in a managed or coordinated manner. Moreover, it has tended to overlook information systems (both paper and electronic) being used by non-statutory agencies in the voluntary community sector (VCS) and private sector as well as information held in various forms by the recipients of care and their informal care networks. Most organisations have amassed a set of systems, often with little coordination of procurement decision-making. (For a discussion of the situation from a general practice information systems perspective, see Sugden *et al.* 2008.) There is now increasing pressure to integrate such systems in localities with existing systems within the organisation (e.g. housing benefit and council tax systems in local government contexts), directly with other organisations (e.g. mental health trust systems in a point-to-point integration for the production of an integrated mental health record) or with a range of other systems (e.g. in the context of partnership working around child protection). The public sector, in particular health and most recently children's services, has seen the locus of control change from locality procured systems to the deployment of a range of nationally procured systems aimed at 'shrink-wrapped' integration within local care situations.

Indeed, for some, the capacity to integrate key systems, in particular integration across platforms (e.g. for single service cross-cutting applications such as SAP) with service-specific applications (e.g. social work records systems) and back-office administrative systems, has been seen as the central agenda for the modernisation of care for older people. The widespread delivery of national systems such as the NHS Spine summary record potentially creates new integration requirements. For many working in IT in the sector (on both the supply and the business requirements side), integration and interoperatability (including standards) remain a, if not the, current focus of attention as the standard response to the 'joining-up' problem.

The only answer, in other words, that currently appears to be in play is 'integration', either 'deep–vertical' or 'broad–horizontal'. However, the who, how and why of the process of integrating and the alternative notions of how services (both organisational and technical) can be coordinated remain relatively unexplored. The problem of integration can be summarised in the question: what else needs to be integrated when we integrate services and information? It is clear that, within the service procurement environment, government policy is aiming to promote a diverse range of service commissioners and service providers in order to deliver the objectives of *personalised* care and *choice*. In order for this to be delivered, a more 'loosely coupled' (Wieck 2001) service environment based on a variety of potential relationships (including services from currently unforeseen providers) needs to be envisaged and subsequently cultivated to support agile responses to both anticipated and emergent care requirements. For this to come into being, a sociotechnical or open systems approach (Wilson *et al.* 2007) to the process of deployment of such service environments needs to take place that explicitly takes into account the relationships between the technical affordances of the information systems (including both paper-based and Web 2.0), disciplinary and interdisciplinary practices and professional, organisational and partnership governance structures.

It seems increasingly clear that the 'market' remains immature where various models of doing business or delivering services (rather than business models in the usual sense) are in play. The diverse sets of values, including modes of value creation, and services that are in play range from the device supplier at one end through the plethora of existing statutory and non-statutory service providers in these areas (who have varying levels of interest in and dependency on the service delivery) to the local vicar and next door neighbour at the other. Only when the local diversity and complexity of roles and relationships begin to be addressed in relation to each other through a process that supports local co-production can we start to 'make sense' of what a national model may look like.

3 Partnership in assessment?

A case study of integrated information sharing

Leigh Keeble, Brian D. Loader
and Michael Hardey

Introduction

The implementation of health and social care policies directed at providing integrated user-centred services for older people remains perhaps the single most important challenge to the modernisation of adult social care in the UK. Research findings, policy reports and government directives have consistently documented the poor quality of services for older people arising from inadequate interagency communication and user–professional relationships that foster dependence (Payne *et al.* 2002). There can be little doubting the magnitude of the task of restructuring differentiated welfare institutions and specialised professional practices that have become so well established. The intention to meet this challenge and drive forward reform, which would instil collaborative working arrangements supported by integrative information systems, was proclaimed by the UK government in a series of influential policy directives. Foremost among these was the *National Service Framework for Older People* (Department of Health 2001a), which introduced the single assessment process (SAP). Significantly, this was quickly followed by the publication of the *Information Strategy for Older People in England* (Department of Health 2002a), which began a new emphasis upon information and communications technologies (ICTs) as an essential means to enable collaborative assessment and joint care provision.

The SAP is intended to be a joint enquiry by those with an interest in the care and support of older people. It is the principal mechanism by which information about the user's social and health condition is drawn together from a variety of professional, agency, familial and community sources to a single point to enable decisions to be made and a course of action to be undertaken. This partnership approach to assessment is designed to both overcome the fragmented investigations and consultations between users and numerous separate agencies and replace them by a collaborative network of providers that places the user at the centre of decision making. Successful implementation of a user-centred partnership such as the SAP is crucially dependent upon developing a commonly accepted information system that facilitates a number of requirements. It should enable the sharing of information, its analysis and interpretation, the communication of knowledge that arises, signal appropriate courses of action, store and archive information to develop a flexible and intelligent knowledge-based system for monitoring and continuous care.

Adult social care is unquestionably an *information-intensive* business requiring enormous amounts of data to be collected from a complex variety of medical and welfare institutions (e.g. hospitals, clinics, laboratories, surgeries) and social and community agents (e.g. housing, voluntary and community groups, social services, carers, community nurses). It should not be surprising, therefore, that ICTs are regarded as a means to both transform service information processing as well as 'informing' and empowering the service user (Emery *et al.* 2002). This restructuring process, which we describe as the *informatisation of adult social care*, is part of the wider agenda to modernise public services (Newman 2001) and restructure welfare relations (Loader 1998).

Information and the nature of its communication are central to the assessment process and the means to integrated service provision. Yet this very primacy also highlights how the processes of design, implementation and adoption of new information systems constitute domains for conflicting visions, interpretations, resistance and opposition. The codification and access to knowledge structure to a significant extent the relations of authority between respective professionals and users of health and social services. To attempt to reconfigure the ownership, flows and barriers to information therefore have important consequences for the self-perceptions and identities of patients, carers, managers and professionals alike. What is too often presented as a simple technical means to improve the efficiency of the system could more accurately be seen as a desire on the part of policy-makers to reinvent the system (Loader 1999).

These tensions between the knowledge-based territories of professional, managerial and user domains are often played out at the frontline of service delivery. The role of street-level bureaucrats such as health care professionals and social workers in influencing the implementation of policies has been a well-documented theme in the academic literature (Prottas 1979; Lipskey 1980). Local implementation of the SAP is significantly influenced by the respective responses to new collaborative working arrangements that arise from introducing integrated information assessment tools. This is especially important for facilitating changes in the relationship between service users and providers that has been a feature of government policy statements. A consumerist emphasis upon patients' charters has been replaced by a rhetoric of 'partnership' that argues for the inclusion of users in the design and negotiation of their assessment. Underpinning this partnership and enabling its integration is the proposed development of fully functioning local electronic information systems (EIS) known as eSAP. This would appear to demand an information system that could be accessed by health and social care practitioners, patients/clients/users or carers,[1] the voluntary and community sector, and also act as a resource for management.

How then are the prospective partners to the SAP responding to these policy visions at the local level? How are local policy-makers and managers interpreting national policy directives for frontline service implementation? What is the perception of health and social care professionals to team working, information sharing and involving users in assessment and delivery? Are EIS tools useable, accessible, reliable and acceptable to the SAP partners? This chapter tries to address these questions by examining the implementation of the SAP in one local area case study that attempted to develop a partnership approach to assessment through integrated teams. It provides a picture of the real life challenges and experiences of dedicated professionals committed to realising the promised benefits of integrated user-centred services outlined in government statements. Strong indications for improvements in assessment and service delivery arising from integrated teamwork and knowledge sharing are clearly evidenced. So too, however, is a message of unrequited receptiveness to these positive lessons from national policy-makers and politicians intent upon permanent public service reinvention.

The case study and method

County Northern is a large mainly rural county with a complex array of organisations and agencies providing health and social care to its population of older people. Statutory social care is provided and delivered across the county by the Social Care and Health Department (SC&HD) of the County Council. In addition, there are seven district or borough councils that are responsible for the delivery of housing services. Health care is provided at the community level though the primary care trusts (PCTs) comprising GPs and community nurses. These public services are supplemented by a range of private organisations, voluntary sector, community and family support networks.

The need to implement the SAP in County Northern provided an important catalyst at a strategic level to address the wider concerns about the quality of services provided to older people and their fragmented nature. Some areas of County Northern had previously established voluntary partnerships between the borough councils, health and social care department and PCTs. The promising results that emerged meant that it was decided to expand this approach across the county through the introduction of additional agency partnerships, which would in turn form the basis for the creation of integrated teams. These teams would be supported in their undertaking of the SAP by an EIS that was an updated version of the existing Social Services Information Database (SSID) system.

During the course of our investigation (2004–6), the county faced two reorganisation challenges that arose from central government directives and had important consequences for the implementation of the SAP. First, in 2003–4, there was a review of local government boundaries. This involved a referendum in the North-east to ascertain the attitude of the population towards the creation of a new regional tier of government to be called the North-east

Assembly. One part of the proposed reorganisation was the dissolution of County Northern and its replacement by three unitary authorities. Despite the fact that no clear support for reorganisation was forthcoming and the county boundaries and role of County Hall was maintained, this process effectively put strategic service planning on hold and delayed the implementation of policy initiatives. Of more significance was the proposal by the Department of Health (DH) to reduce the number of PCTs in England from 303 to 152 with the anticipated changes taking place by October 2006. PCTs would become patient-centred and commissioning-led organisations (Department of Health 2005a). Following a period of consultation, it was announced in the summer of 2006 that the five existing PCTs in the county would be merged into one covering the whole of the county. As we shall see, these policy directives had a significant effect upon the introduction of the SAP and the efficacy of integrated working practices.

The investigation itself consisted of a mixture of forty-two interviews with managers and service professionals, twelve focus groups with service users and access to policy documentation, all of which was undertaken between July 2004 and October 2006. While we considered county-wide strategic policy, our main focus was an in-depth analysis of one partnership area. Meadowfield was one of the earliest and therefore offered the richest findings for our investigation.

Towards integrated e-assessment?

Building upon the previous successful project initiatives, the development of integrated health and social care service provision to older people in County Northern was pursued on the basis of voluntary partnerships between borough councils, health and social care departments and PCTs. This was facilitated in part by coterminous boundaries shared by the respective agencies. An evaluation of the early stages of the Meadowfield partnership undertaken in July 2004 described it as a high-performing collaboration. Such perceived progress understandably made these partnerships an ideal bedrock upon which to further develop integrated working practices across the county as a whole. Consequently, it was decided to introduce agency partnerships in all five districts in the county. During the course of our investigation, the successful establishment of partnerships was mixed, with most development occurring in the pilot area of Meadowfield, which was the predominant focus of our research.

The plan in Meadowfield was to have five integrated locality teams employing around thirty to forty staff by the end of April 2005. It is at this service level that the SAP comes into operation as the primary means of integrating social workers, community nurses and housing officers. Moreover, the response of frontline staff to partnership working through the adoption of the SAP and ICTs was always going to be crucial for the implementation and successful working of the integrated teams. While integration of care was the avowed objective, what emerged from the data is a theme constructed around 'professional territories' and the challenges to their permeability. These territories can be defined as including both 'professional cultures' (e.g. difference in training, role and so forth between social workers and nurses) and areas of practice. It is therefore appropriate to examine the experiences and perceptions of the main occupational groups involved in the integration process.

1 Social workers

The particular EIS platform chosen by the county to support the SAP and adopted for use by the integrated team that participated in this case study was an adapted version of an established SSID. The interface of this system provides both a multichoice 'tick box' feature together with open boxes providing space for practitioners to include narrative material. Thus it is designed to support a standardised assessment comprising information intended to identify the possible health, social and housing needs of the user at a single point of data entry. While the whole assessment procedure required all the fields to be completed, it is also designed to be flexible. Social workers had become familiar with SSIDs, and SAP was essentially layered on top of SSID. During a consultation process, it was found that health staff required a more structured approach to the assessment than social workers who favoured a more discursive approach. This reflects the way in which, for social workers, there can be a therapeutic dimension to a consultation with a client. The traditionally more bodily concerns of health practitioners can be usefully captured in a checklist of items that ensure the user's health has been properly assessed. The SAP tool was consequently designed to be more prescriptive, with a range of headings and a number of tick box options under those headings. Space was also provided for more qualitative information or comments. However, the form could be completed with little narrative information. Similar design compromises have been reported in other areas (Powell *et al.* 2007).

The apparent loss of significance of narrative material under SAP enabled social workers who had reservations to the changes under way to argue that this amounted to what they describe as deskilling. A Service Development Officer explained the situation: ' ... we've just had 117 social workers sign a petition to say they don't like SAP and they think its wrong ... and it's deskilling them'.

The perceived professional deskilling appeared to focus around two dimensions of the SAP. First, the social workers regarded the process of inputting data as akin to 'clinical' box ticking or what several described as the 'ticky box syndrome'. Second, the joint working arrangements were requiring social workers to undertake what they regarded as 'health' assessments as well as the 'social' assessments for which they saw themselves as professionally qualified. These two factors raised issues for the social workers about how the SAP tool may act to reshape their professional practice and influence trust relationships between themselves and the service users.

What the social workers are really naffed off about is the fact that [SAP's] taken away what they did. We've given them this new tool they don't have a choice but, as their employers we can do that, but the NHS staff are all supposed to use the same tool and input information, they don't do anything like the same level. So the social workers feel it is an added burden on them having to provide information which is not just their responsibility and they are right.

SC&HD, Service Development Officer

This concurred with observations made by social workers that the interview time with older service users was increasingly shaped by what they regarded as 'data capture', which was replacing what they saw as a more 'sensitive' if not therapeutic interaction and appraisal of the users' needs (cf. Smale *et al.* 1993). Indeed, disaffected social workers argued that the 'data collection' was not important for the user but, rather, to 'feed the beast with data that someone else will use'. Underwriting divisions among practitioners are different models of users. Health professionals were essentially following a medically orientated approach, while social workers were orientated towards a therapeutic enabling model.

The clash of professional cultures manifest in the reaction of some social workers became a major hurdle that managers stated they had to overcome. Indeed, such was the strength of feeling among social workers in a neighbouring area that a senior manger noted that a decision had been taken to 'follow' the lead taken by other areas in relation to SAP by pursuing a 'wait and see' approach. However, County Northern was committed to change and, as a Divisional Commissioning Manager explained, there was an acknowledgement of the issues highlighted by social workers:

… social workers having to ask questions about health promotion. I mean they absolutely hate it, not all of them but the vast majority of them, they can't get their heads around why they have to enquire about people's blood pressure, smoking, drinking, diet, exercise, all of those things.

At management level, there was the expectation that, once integrated teams were established, there would be a greater recognition of the role and relevance of other practitioners involved in the delivery of care:

Now in some of the integrated teams it's beginning to make a bit more sense because they sit next to the nurses and they might begin to understand it and the nurse will say we'll send them to the smoking cessation clinic or something, you know, but a lot of them don't like it, not comfortable with it. So on the one hand we're deskilling them, on the other hand they're being stretched beyond their training, we're turning them into nurses.

Despite the concerns and resistances noted above, by the final phase of interviews, the experience of working within an integrated team is summed up by one social worker who explained:

> The integrated team is district nurses, social workers, housing, these kind of people all work together under the same roof. The single assessment process is done once and all details put onto a computer. I spoke to housing and a social worker and they found that the benefits were that instead of coming into the office and having to get the diary out to organise things, we are now all under one roof. The process is much quicker. All the details are here and up to date.

There is a caveat here that those social workers (and other practitioners) who were resistant to such working arrangements may have chosen to move to other posts or areas close by where implementation had taken a different course.

2 Community nurses

Tension between different professional cultures has been noted elsewhere (e.g. Postle 2002). However, these tensions were largely played out between practitioners and management rather than between social workers and community nurses or housing staff. An integrated team manager put this rather well when stating that 'the social workers all think it [SAP] is all health dominated, the nurses think it's all social care'. As noted above, some social workers believed that 'health' was gaining ground over social care in the delivery of care to older people. There was little evidence to suggest that nurses held this view. Indeed, there was recognition by nurses that they had worked in something of a 'health silo' that militated against good working relationships and the sharing of information with others:

> ... in the past we could barely see a Social Worker face to face and you never had any contact with them. Now [following integration] we have face to face contact and we know more about each other's position and role than ever before and I know what a Housing person can do for me and so on. I think that it would be harder to continue working how we did before.
> Community nurse

The aforementioned concerns expressed by frontline staff about the implications for their working practices and professional identity as a consequence of SAP and ICT arrangements provided challenges to implementing integrated teams. A community partnership manager based in Meadowfield gives an indication of the tense working environment in the early stages of integration.

> I came from a social care background at a very difficult time because of change and it was a huge learning curve for me and a very negative time

for me, because there were a lot of staff that were very much against integration, who did not want to go into integrated teams of social care practitioners.

Despite these tribulations, however, analysis based on the last phase of interviews revealed a picture of the Meadowfield integrated team beginning to develop a shared working relationship. Even from the outset, the value of collaborative arrangements was learnt.

> The very first day that the team went live there was a referral from one of the GP practices that was complex, it needed involvement by the nursing services, it needed involvement by social workers and on this occasion also needed involvement by the supporting housing officer. I think from day one the penny dropped, that the three agencies working that closely together, within a matter of hours real progress had been made with that one individual case and I really do believe that from that point on, you know, things changed.
>
> Community partnership manager

Meadowfield had an advantage over other districts in that it was seen by County Northern as something of a 'demonstrator' group and had a very experienced community partnership manager as the lead. A theme that emerged from the analysis of the last phase of interviews with both frontline staff and managers was the importance of the commitment of management to ICTs and integration:

> The strength of the partnership is based on key personalities (in the Borough Council, PCT and Social Care and Health) and those three senior people drove this forward and it worked because of that. That partnership works with that commitment. If one was to leave, or there was external pressure then that could break down.
>
> Manager of integration, PCT

A significant factor that frontline staff and management identified as fostering information sharing was the physical co-location of the integrated team on one site:

> … it helps that the team's all in the same area because we bat things off each other, you know, I mean one can be talking about a patient in one room and somebody else will say 'Oh well I've been there lately' and, you know, and that's how it works with the integration, so it's ideal.
>
> Community nurse

> In terms of being co-located I think for the client it is definitely better. How many times if someone has a housing problem are you told that 'you

need to speak to my social worker, they've got all the details'? You try to ring the social worker, the social worker is out on a visit, you can't get hold of them, so then it goes into a next day.

Housing support officer

The link between co-location and its ability to facilitate higher trust relationships through face-to-face contact, quicker responses to queries, shared information and greater understanding between the frontline team was also identified as being important for successful integration. The key dimensions of familiarity and trust are identified by a community partnership manager:

I think that the most important thing is for everyone to trust each other. It has never been a problem here. We respect each other and there has been a willingness to work with one another here. That comes a lot from being in the same place and we want to make each other's jobs easier and that benefits the clients. You don't have to wait for days for response from colleagues. I don't buy the virtual integration. There are so many opportunities to get instant advice and be face to face and that's preferable to virtual contact.

It is instructive to compare the apprehension about integration that was common among social workers noted earlier and the comment below from a social worker situated within the team:

My role here is what may be called a Social Worker, but is more about a care commissioner co-ordinator. There's no lead agency. We will liaise with nursing, it's all mixed in. It's more about being fluid. I have to do a lot more thinking outside the box. Here boundaries are blurred. For example this morning I was looking at getting a gentleman home who is diabetic, and is not eating. I need to make sure that he has a carer there to make sure that he gets his insulin and is taking food. So there is a lot of blurring there, it may be a medical need but there is a social need there as well, to ensure that he can be maintained at home.

It would be wrong to imply that the above is representative, but this sense of 'blurring' as opposed to 'de-skilling' marks a potentially significant shift in the stance of practitioners. Crucial to this development was both the co-location of the professionals, which assisted deliberation, and the access to data afforded by the EIS.

Involving the users in assessment

A fully integrated SAP, as stated at the outset, places the user at the centre of the process and delivery. While the partnerships and integrated teams discussed so far suggest the potential to reconfigure territories of care, our investigation was also concerned to see how user-centred assessment could be introduced. In relation to the development of the EIS, one might expect that a user-centred approach would embrace a co-construction or mutual shaping of the technology (Bijker 1995; Oudshoorn & Pinch 2005). However, the opportunity to involve users more directly in the design and development of the EIS was severely circumscribed at the outset by the pragmatic decision to adapt the existing SSIDs to the new demands of SAP and integration. As we could find no evidence for the inclusion of older people in any system design exercises or of any user modelling within the various innovations to EIS, this section focuses on the *experiences* of using the system provided. We consider first the views of older people derived from a series of focus groups and, again, these are illustrated by extracts from these data. This is followed by the perceptions of the frontline staff and management to user-centred service delivery.

1 Users' perspective

The initial responses from the users expressed a traditional understanding of the expert/user relationship where the former acts as a gatekeeper to services and interventions (Parsons 1951). Interestingly, however, users were becoming aware of a change in attitude on the part of professionals, as one person explained:

> ... now then this is a point that we brought up right, what 15 year ago even. Doctors were treated as Gods, and the nurses that came in to see you, and the midwife that came in to see you at a home birth were helpers of God. That system has gone now. At least it should have gone by now and some of the younger doctors are coming in with a new attitude ...

The moves to 'expert patients', 'user-centredness' and 'partnerships' in care have been sufficiently established to have become embedded in the training of health and social care professionals and form part of the expectations of accrediting bodies. Users are now established as active participants in their care across the health and welfare service. Enhanced choice through the negotiation of assessments and other mechanisms delivers personalised care that fosters feelings of independence and empowerment (Leadbeater 2004). Information is central to the development of personalised care as it forms the basis for choices. However, while SAP and other strategies effectively capture information, choice is more problematic as it assumes that all parties have both the information and the experiences on which to base decisions. Whatever the aspirations to equality in expert/user relationships and despite significant policies such as direct payments, the practitioner retains knowledge (both practice-based and tacit information about local resources and gatekeepers) and can exercise discretion about choices. Moreover, as noted earlier, the generation of older people who are subject to this research express largely deferential views about the qualities of practitioners in whom they want to invest trust. However, within County Northern, practitioners remain 'experts' whom older people view as a scarce resource they should not 'trouble' or call upon too much. One participant explained:

> All I know over the years are that social workers are swamped with work, have too many clients so they can't handle any new work …

This sense of 'swamped' related to how some older people viewed practitioners. They argued that 'people are too proud' to either take up services that they were entitled to or attempt to find information that was not provided by those immediately engaged in their care. Significantly, this discourse was usually phrased in terms of 'others' displaying this degree to deference to professionals.

Analysis of focus group data produced a division between those who were against wanting to know what was on their records and others who wanted some access. However, a distinction may need to be made between detailed medical records and broader instruments such as SAP. Medical records prompted a rather different debate that rotated around the desire (or not) to know whether an illness was terminal or not. No one reported that they had seen such records, although some had seen care plans.

Concern was expressed about the accuracy of information that was retained by health and social services rather than an individual's direct access to such material. The comment below sums up the position:

> … ignorance is bliss, but I would want to know what has been written about me and is it accurate. I don't know how I would know that it was accurate. I would want to know that what was there was accurate.

One person explained that 'we need to know so we can challenge the information'. Yet users were also worried about their ability to understand such information. A retired nurse summed this position up:

> I think that is dangerous, as the medical profession use abbreviated language that could be misinterpreted and taken the wrong way. You are at liberty now to see the letters if you want. Quite frankly having seen some of these reports, when it was my job and extracting things, I don't think that I would want to know everything that they had written. Seriously I don't think that I would want to know everything that is going on in my insides, I am happy as I am and they can keep it between medical professionals.

Some users were worried that practitioners may not have sufficient access to information. As one explained:

I think the professionals ... should have more information to be able to give it out to you, I mean it just keeps going round and round in circles doesn't it all the time, there's not enough information anywhere.

A further vignette was designed to explore whether those who had experienced integrated teams felt it changed the delivery of services to them. Again, there was a division of opinion here that can be illustrated by the following extract:

> ... the government's ideas about single assessment aren't realistic like this when there isn't the money in the system to pay for the recommendations. I think we're quite lucky that the integrated team ... is starting to really show that they can deliver information or can deliver services quite quickly. You ... fill in one form and have one visit and it goes back to a team and the team consists of health, social services, housing and other I think currently occupational therapists.

2 Frontline staff and user-centred assessment

Interviews with frontline staff revealed a division of opinion between community nurses and the social workers, with the former being more reticent about user access to their information than the latter. The comments by community staff nurses reproduced below are indicative:

> I don't think that patients should have access to the kind of information on SSID.
>
> Patients? Oh no. I would not be happy about that. I suppose that they are entitled to see their own medical records, but you would have to think more carefully about what kind of information would be on there. At the moment it is aimed at the professionals reading each other's information.

Social workers were more sympathetic to user access and sometimes positively advocated wider online access to service user information by the users themselves:

> It's about democratising. Saying these are your notes, not the GP's, not mine or social services, but your notes and here they are. So yes why not do that after all the price of computers is falling.

Indeed, as the following quote suggests, some social workers were advocates of practices that would make users more informed:

> I do enjoy going out and talking to informed people. It makes our job easier. The individual knows what the issues are and what they want. Great just sign. It makes my job easier and they are offering me informed opinion and that's great.

This divergence between health and social care practitioners again reflects different professional territories and practices. Health care information, symbolised by patient notes, has historically been seen as 'confidential' and 'sensitive'. Moreover, medical expertise is bound to an abstract system that uses a language and concepts that may require a degree of interpretation if data are reconfigured from an expert/expert to an expert/user interface. In effect, this act of interpretation remains central to the practitioner/user relationship. In addition, as noted above, older people may not necessarily desire full disclosure of their medical records. Social workers' claims to expertise have a different and more narrative basis (see tensions over the SAP form noted earlier) that is combined with a therapeutic view of the expert/user encounter. To put it simply, social work cannot have recourse to the body as a source of knowledge and so is reliant on some degree of communicative collaboration with users.

3 Management and user-centred services

Analysis of the interviews with managers revealed a desire to emphasise the importance of the individual user to assessment procedures and service delivery. However, this was frequently balanced by a sceptical view about meeting the policy objective of achieving a user-led approach. Concerns focused upon the complexity of the system and the ability of users to find their way around it.

> Well you're not talking about user-centred services. They're talking about user-led services aren't they? They're commissioning a patient-led NHS and the choice agenda and it's completely baffling for professionals, so what it's like if you are 75 I can't actually imagine ... I just think it's so confusing really. So nice in theory but chaotic to implement.
>
> Director of integration, PCT

There was also awareness by some interviewees that the more socially advantaged users may have a competitive advantage over others in using the system. In a welfare service with an ethos of providing services according to assessed needs, this raised concerns over equitable access. User-centred driven services, which might increasingly be based upon the ability to understand and navigate EIS in order to access services and resources, may lead to an uneven distribution of provision based upon networking confidence rather than assessed need. Consequently, it was thought that it might be necessary to ensure that those more likely to be excluded would be provided with effective support:

> ... that's the worry about the choice agenda because you've got to be intelligent and articulate really to use the system to your advantage. I think it's, you know, vulnerable groups who need guiding through the system, you've got to have a particular arrangement to help those people.

Managing the implementation of SAP

The introduction of SAP and attendant technologies was framed by broad government implementation guidelines that were intended to facilitate approaches that could flexibly take account of local needs and past histories. During the research, a new initiative that would result in an integrated children's record system and electronic care record was announced (Department of Health 2003, 2004b). This provided a revealing opportunity for managers to compare the children's approach to developing an integrated EIS with that previously adopted for older people:

> If you look at the children's agenda there's some big initiatives running there round integrated children's system and common assessment framework where the government have basically said there's the documentation and the guidance with it, get on and implement it. If you want to add a few things in locally, fair enough, but essentially one set of documentation for the whole of the country, that's good practice, that's what you should be doing. For the single assessment, for some reason, they accredited completely different tools and even then said, as long as most agencies sign up locally you can do your own as well. So I think there's something like 20 different tools actually in use across the whole of the country for single assessment which is barmy, for want of a better expression, and I think it would be much more appreciated if they said look I know there's local needs and local circumstances but essentially that's the tool you use, if you want to add to it feel free, but that's the tool you use, and I think it would have been a much more successful project if they'd done that.
>
> SC&HD, Information and communications manager

Others echoed this view, and it might be acknowledged that the children's initiative strategy may have been influenced by experiences with the older people's programme.

What were identified as 'territories of care' that involve organisations and geographical barriers to integration and information exchange were also identified as a fetter upon developing a comprehensive EIS. The following remark nicely indicates the challenges of sharing information between organisations in different locations where their systems are incompatible:

> Even now in Northern and East and North Wells and Haverpool they're working on converging the three completely separate tools into one common tool but South Wells will still be using a different one and probably Southumbria will be. So even though we're trying to do things locally to get a single tool, it means that when we sort of exchange information with our partners in other patches they're probably using a different tool altogether which just adds to the difficulty.
>
> SC&HD, Service development officer

Without an agreed national EIS that would enable information sharing across geographical, organisational and professional territories, such barriers are likely to continue to provide persistent challenges to the implementation of SAP.

By far the most significant concern to managers, however, was what we describe as *policy initiative fatigue* and the demands it made upon both providing a coordinated response and the morale of staff. We use the term *policy initiative fatigue* to refer to a policy environment that is perceived to be in a constant state of change, providing frequent central directives for implementation by local agents, which makes integrated strategic planning and operational delivery very challenging. This flow of policy directives from government departments raised a number of issues from the respondents that are exemplified by the selected quotations from the interview data. First was a frustration about the seemingly poor level of compatibility between policy objectives:

> I think policy is not sufficiently thought through so you get lots of conflicting policy initiatives. So [for example] integration and choice and competition don't actually all fit together so there's lots of conflicting policy agendas ... I read something ... [which] said there was something like ... 200,000 pages of new policy that NHS managers have had to implement in the past year ... You just think no wonder we feel ... it is very, very difficult. I think a lot of it's well intentioned; it just feels like different parts of the department don't speak to each other really.
>
> Director, PCT

An environment of policy change is a common context for people operating at senior level in public sector agencies. However, from the analysis of interview data across all phases of the study, it was evident that senior managers in particular believed that they were having to work in the context of an unusually high number of government initiatives and other actual and potential changes to their situation. Working in this environment raised concerns about becoming distracted from service delivery. One director explained the situations thus:

> Well we're trying to deal with so many [policy directives] at the same time that inevitably you just end up feeling like you're feeding the beast and you're not really making genuine improvements in services for patients ... There are some helpful policy initiatives but I don't think there's enough joining up of things in particular.
>
> Director, PCT

In effect, the need to respond quickly to potential or actual policy and consequent organisational changes took resources away from ongoing longer term projects such as service integration and EIS development. As mentioned at the beginning, in the course of the research, PCTs in County Northern were reduced from five to one covering the whole county. This was not only regarded as deleterious to staff morale, but was also seen to undermine existing local moves to integration and SAP:

> One thing that we did not do was to put forward a model that would be future proof. The risk of government review has been tested because of health service reform. With the changes in the PCTs I doubt that people at a senior level are going to agree to develop integrated teams. At this stage you cannot articulate the state of money. You can show that there are a set of costs. Changes to PCTs could kill integration. This is critical to the services and they may say that the PCT future is as a commissioning body and there may not be room for integrated teams and the delivery arm. Maybe you have to step outside of this and deliver services in a different way. Because it's voluntary what's happening with external pressure could kill it.
>
> Head of neighbourhood service, Borough council

The extract above reflects two significant themes evident from interviews with managers at all levels. First, that financial planning was exacerbated due to uncertainties with regard to organisational responsibilities and, second, that priorities were subject to change so that initiatives such as integration may suffer in the face of new agendas. The quotation below neatly captures what some described as 'frustration' with the flow of new initiatives:

> ... the integration process over in Eastwold ... sort of almost came to a halt as soon as the patient led commissioning came onto [the agenda] ... The new White Paper's come out ... and says the Meadowfield model is an area of good practice and yet ... there are lots of areas of change being driven by central government policy that takes you down a different route.
>
> SC&HD, Service development office

> ... the amount of time it takes just to build up your systems, your network, your structures and, you know, we're really not even there yet to be honest, we're just at the point where we're getting the structure fit for purpose and then we're changing.
>
> Director, PCT

Given the prominent role of the PCTs in the formation of integrated teams, this reorganisation raised questions about the future of the local teams. At the time of the last phase of interviews, no decision as to the future of the PCTs had been announced, so funding decisions and posts had been frozen.

Conclusions

Case studies of implementation such as this one can only provide a limited and partial view of a complex policy development (Yin 2003). Nonetheless, they are valuable for foregrounding some significant issues and providing nuanced critical feedback from the ground level, which can inform policy deliberation higher up. In this case, some very positive indications of effective integrated team working based upon a combination of physical co-location and a shared EIS suggest that opportunities for improved health and social care services for older people could be developed more widely.

Some initial resistance to the implementation of integration and ICTs by frontline staff was overcome by training and the experience of working within an integrated team. This fostered cooperation and trust across professional territories. Physical co-location of the integrated team did much to promote this culture as well as the common use of the EIS framework and SAP tool. For managers, the EIS provided the potential to view and manage current demands made on human and material resources and, consequently, contributed to more responsive decision-making based upon a broader conception of user needs. This affirms that training and support for frontline staff when implementing new information systems and working practices foster effective working relationships and cannot be underemphasised. Furthermore, it signifies that co-location has benefits in promoting collaboration across professional territories and effective team working (e.g. joint problem solving, enhanced response times and mutual understanding).

User engagement with EIS, however, continued to be mediated by practitioners and thereby helped to reinforce the practitioner/user relationship, which significantly limits user choice. This is unlikely to change with the implementation of eSAP, and the presence of a laptop may instead enhance the sense of expertise invested by older people in practitioners. Users appear to be more marginalised in the design and implementation of the EIS than policies and documentation suggested when the research project was commenced. Older people were concerned that information about them should be accurate and accessible to those who delivered service to them. However, they had no sense of 'ownership' of such information, which they saw as compiled by and situated in the domain of practitioners. It is desirable to enable users to have a sense of ownership of such information and to provide them with direct access to information so that they can, for example, update information or check for accuracy. Those older people who have become familiar with ICTs (e.g. through email, arranging holidays, purchasing books, etc.) may increasingly come to expect such access. By enabling users to directly connect to a health and social care EIS, a new conduit for the sharing of information and decisions could be opened. This potentially offers considerable cost savings in terms of time and human resources compared with face-to-face interactions.

Despite the encouraging developments towards integrated working and the commitment of the professionals and managers involved in the implementation of the SAP, a striking feature of the investigation was the identification of an almost Sisyphean attitude that the task could never be completed in the face of policy flux and overload. The constant flow of policy directives from government departments and the perceived incompatibility of many of these objectives combined to provide a picture of uncoordinated and disjointed policy-making leading to policy initiative fatigue at the ground level. This was seen as particularly frustrating by local managers and frontline staff in a situation where they believed real progress was being made towards realising integration and partnership working. It may be important therefore that, in considering modernisation policies which have ambitious transforming objectives, the negative consequences of policy initiative fatigue upon the managers and staff responsible for implementation should be an essential component of the initial strategic risk assessment of such policies.

Finally, the experience of modifying an existing local information database care system to support partnership and user-centred delivery foregrounds many of the challenges to integration. Our research established that the practitioners and managers both wanted a more prescribed format that would be nationally compatible and enable cross-boundary flows of data and also valued the existing system and wanted to expand it to encompass health records. Such an expansion raises the prospect of extending the assessment procedure still further and would need careful design and implementation. The desire for an integration tool that both provides national health and social care data and is sufficiently flexible to allow local agency, service user and professional authorship makes this a very challenging environment within which to develop eSAP. It suggests a hybrid approach combining nationally set standards facilitating interoperability but enabling partnerships of practitioners, agencies and users to be involved in the design of innovative applications at the local level. At the time of writing, the potential of eSAP to realise such a hybrid option has yet to be proven.

Notes

1 In this chapter, 'users', 'carer' and 'patients' will be used interchangeably.

Part II

User-centred assessment and autonomy

4 Perspectives on telecare

Implications for autonomy, support and social inclusion

*John Percival, Julienne Hanson
and Dorota Osipovič*

Introduction

A significant government effort is underway to make supportive technology services available in the homes of people who might otherwise require institutional care (Department of Health 2002b; King's Fund 2006), through the provision to all local authorities of preventative technology grants totalling around £80 million (Lyall 2005). This technology and the support staff involved is known generically as telecare, a service that delivers care to a user's own home through the provision of information and communications technology (ICT) (Audit Commission 2004b). Telecare can provide virtual interaction with health and social care practitioners as well as close monitoring, through the installation of home-based sensors, of an individual's activities of daily living. These monitoring sensors take two different forms: 'active' monitors, including food detectors and blood pressure monitors, which provide real time responses to environmental or biological changes, and 'passive' lifestyle monitors, in the form of strategically placed sensors that, over time, gather and analyse an individual's domestic routines and behaviour, so as to raise alerts when unusual and worrying changes take place. Telecare therefore includes a preventative element of support that improves upon the basic community alarm system (Brownsell 2000), which has over past decades enabled people to activate a radio pendant or cord switch to raise assistance if in difficulties, a system popular in sheltered housing schemes.

Ambitious claims are often made for telecare, and supporters of the industry argue that, as well as equipment and support, telecare offers dignity and independence (TSA 2007). However, there is a lack of good-quality research about telecare's effectiveness (Hailey *et al.* 2002; Whitten & Richardson 2002). In particular, few studies present the views or experiences of telecare users or potential users (Sixsmith & Sixsmith 2000; Levy *et al.* 2003), and there is little empirical evidence on the ways in which older people use assistive technology (Gann *et al.* 2000). Furthermore, user-focused studies have tended to elicit the views of people living in sheltered housing, where residents already have access to a community alarm system and may therefore be more receptive to telecare. Studies have insufficiently explored telecare's potential with regard to the majority of the older population who live in mainstream housing, who may lack support and social inclusion (Fisk 2003). As a result, relatively little is known about the views and preferences of key stakeholders: potential service users living in ordinary housing, family members who have support responsibilities and care staff based in the community. This chapter and the research[1] upon which it is based seek to widen the debate by providing information that details the potential benefits as well as the limitations of telecare, from a range of perspectives. Discussion begins with an account of research participants' attitudes towards the sort of technology encompassed by telecare and their suggestions for further innovation. This is followed by an analysis of topics that emerged throughout our research, which include the importance of tailoring and targeting telecare services, issues of confidentiality and surveillance, the question of virtual care and social inclusion and, lastly, implications for integrating and resourcing telecare. Before the discussion, we present a brief account of our research methods.

Methodology

The first phase of our research involved convening a series of twenty-two focus group discussions in Plymouth, South Buckinghamshire and Barnsley: ten groups with older people, five with informal carers and seven with relevant professionals. The regional spread of the numbers involved is shown in Table 4.1.

The aim of the focus group discussions was to introduce, for those with little prior knowledge, the concept and details of telecare services and to explore participants' views and opinions, through discussion of various case scenarios. None of the older participants had experience of telecare services, and few of the professionals in the groups had yet embarked on operationalising telecare services. Professional participants represented health, housing and social care agencies, and their affiliation by region is represented in Table 4.2. Further details of how we established this phase of our research have been published previously (Percival & Hanson 2006).

The second phase of our research centred on a pilot project based at a sheltered housing scheme for people with sight loss in Plymouth. Six older tenants agreed to the installation of telecare devices and, over an 11-month period, their experiences were monitored and evaluated by way of regular individual interviews. Table 4.3 presents the characteristics of each of these pilot project participants and the sensors installed.

The equipment installed in each of the participants' flats included a fall detector and an average of fifteen lifestyle monitoring sensors, including passive infrared movement detectors (PIRs), bed occupancy sensors, bed epilepsy sensors, chair occupancy sensors, electric usage sensors (e.g. placed on a TV, kettle or oven) and door contact sensors (placed on wardrobes, fridge-freezers, kitchen cupboards, bathroom cupboards and front doors). In addition, two participants had 'talking' blood pressure monitors. The lifestyle monitoring

Table 4.1 Sample numbers by region

	Older people	Carers	Professionals
Plymouth	31	17	15
S. Bucks	25	27	13
Barnsley/Rotherham	36	11	11
Total	92	55	39

Table 4.2 Professional affiliation by region

Sector	Plymouth	S. Bucks	Barnsley
Health	3	4	5
SSD	3	6	3
LA housing	1	0	2
H Assoc./Trust	4	2	0
Vol. agency	4	1	1
Total	15	13	11

Note: SSD, Social Services Department; LA, local authority; H Assoc., housing association; Vol., voluntary.

sensors provide constant passive monitoring of the domestic environment in order to learn people's normal daily routines and activities and then to recognise and track significant deviations from this norm and alert carers if required. In our project, data derived from the lifestyle monitoring sensors were used for academic purposes, as information for researchers to aggregate and interpret, rather than as a means of obtaining practical support. All participants were made aware of this fact at the beginning of the project. Interpretation of this lifestyle monitoring data is ongoing, and no firm conclusions have yet been reached. This chapter does, however, discuss important issues arising from participants' experiences of learning about and having telecare devices placed in their homes. These issues, together with those raised by the focus group participants, are conflated in this chapter in order to provide a discussion of key themes that emerged across both phases of the research: themes of autonomy, support and social inclusion.

In order to develop these themes in a focused and accessible way, we briefly present Nielsen's model of system acceptability and usability (Nielsen 1993), as adapted by Emery (2001: 45), who reports on a telecare initiative with regard to carers of older people. In this context, usability of technology is understood by paying attention to user acceptance (desire to use the system again and comfort in doing so), social acceptability (related to users' values and beliefs), utility (centres on the benefits experienced by the user) and usability (characteristics of learnability, efficiency, sequences that are memorable, avoidance of errors and satisfaction). We have referred to these categories, both to marshal salient themes arising from focus groups (as indicated in Table 4.4) and to help integrate relevant aspects of this useful model with our discussion.

Table 4.3 Pilot project participant characteristics and sensors installed

Pseudonym of participant	Age (years)	Household composition	Health conditions	Installed sensors
Mrs Adams	80	One person household	Sight loss, hypertension, diabetes	Bed, chair, door, electrical, movement
Mrs Bishop	68	Married couple household	Sight loss, hypertension	Door, electrical, movement
Miss Evans	84	One person household	Sight loss, hearing impairment, coronary heart disease, epilepsy	Bed, chair, door, electrical, movement
Mr Gibson	82	One person household	Sight loss, hypertension, diabetes, cancer	Bed, door, electrical, movement
Mr Heaton	47	One person household	Sight loss, cerebral palsy, hypertension	Door, electrical, movement
Mrs Jenkins	84	One person household	Diabetes, coronary heart disease	Bed, chair, door, electrical, movement

Table 4.4 Nielsen's (1993) categories of system acceptability and related focus group themes

Nielsen's category of model acceptability	Corresponding theme(s) from focus groups
Social acceptability	Personal preferences, choice, privacy
User acceptance	Tailored service, availability of support
Usability	Understandable technology, ease of use, reliability
Utility	Control, security, safety, social inclusion

Attitudes towards telecare technology and indicators for user acceptability

Many of the focus group participants spoke favourably of the potential preventative benefits of telecare devices, such as fall detectors, blood pressure monitors, flood detectors and automatic sensor lights, which could give older people and informal carers 'peace of mind'. Informal carers were vocal in praising technology that enables any changes in activity and possible dangers to be noticed straightaway and which can prompt an individual in certain circumstances, for example if memory retention is a problem. Informal carers also pointed out that telecare monitoring devices can give a more accurate account of an individual's activities of daily living than the subject him or herself, as people sometimes deny their deterioration, an issue we return to later. One public sector online news site (24dash 2007) cites the case of an older woman who was not taking her medication properly, which resulted in frequent visits by her daughter to hand deliver all medication. The situation improved when a medication dispenser linked to a Lifeline home unit was installed, which subsequently provided the correct doses and alerted the daughter if the tablets had not been taken.

The talking blood pressure monitor was particularly valued by the visually impaired participants in our pilot project, who praised the design features that made this device interactive, responsive and easy to use, putting the control of the device entirely in the hands of the service user and leading to a personal sense of empowerment. In general, the pilot project participants advocated that sensors should provide voice prompts and verbal feedback rather than visual prompt and cues, which are of little help to people with sight loss. However, some participants questioned the suitability of voice prompts for those who are hard of hearing, who typically take out their hearing aids at night. If voice prompts are made loud to compensate, this could disturb neighbours, indicating that the technology has to be evaluated in respect of its suitability in the context of the individual's immediate environment. In addition, there was a professional viewpoint that ICT, such as video conferencing, could allow ready access to a client and therefore help to reassure health or social care practitioners about that individual's well-being.

Telecare's potential for providing improvements in safety for people at home is clearly important, as indicated by the creative thinking of our focus group lay participants, who made suggestions for devices that they thought should be prototyped and which we represent in Table 4.5.

Table 4.5 Participants' additional suggestions for useful devices

Type of device	Attributes
Body temperature monitor	Checks for hypothermia
Water temperature control	Reduce risk of scalding Reduce risk of hypothermia
Voice prompts	Remind to take medication
Interactive blood pressure monitor	Warning given if blood pressure rising
Fall detector fitted to wrist/ankle	Discrete, comfortable, secure
Wandering monitor at window	May prevent exit by person with dementia
Coded button door release	May prevent exit by person with dementia
Tracking device (aesthetically designed and lightweight)	Easier location of wanderer
'Remote' community alarm	User can tell staff if lost

According to our interviewees, the usability of a piece of technology is contingent on its design, sensitivity, reliability and, ultimately, the user's peace of mind. Design was a significant factor in discussions and application of the fall detector. In theory, the fall detector ticked the right boxes, as it can raise alerts when a person is not able to do so following a fall. In practice, our pilot participants found the device to be bulky and inconvenient to wear. Participants also criticised the design of chair sensors that could not be fitted to recliner chairs. Devices that are hypersensitive also affect people's perceptions of usability and, paradoxically, their sense of security, a point raised in connection with the fall detector, which can raise an alert even if accidentally dropped. The prospect of accidental but repeated call-out of staff responding to false alarms worries older people, who fear that this may endanger their relationship with staff and lead to a call for the older person's removal to institutional care. Indeed, technology that is seen as too sensitive or unreliable may be rejected by older people (Pagnell *et al.* 2000; Bowes & McColgan 2003; King 2004).

Reliability becomes an issue when people experience a fault, either because a device's batteries have failed or because the alert triggered by a device is attributed to the wrong service user, events that affected participants during the pilot phase of our research. Behind such concerns is the need for clarification about who would be responsible for servicing the technology, how its effectiveness would be monitored and who would respond when there are problems or when a device needs to be reset after a shut-down, such as would occur when the gas supply is automatically turned off.

At the heart of the issue of usability, and central to much of our discussion of telecare, is the need for technological support services that are individually tailored, so as to meet personal requirements, and are properly targeted at those who need and want the service.

Tailoring and targeting telecare

Personal interest and subjective need affect attitudes to and user acceptance of telecare. Some pilot participants engaged in the project because of their personal enthusiasm for technology, while others were more reticent or disinclined to be involved through aversion or unease with new technologies. For example, some pilot participants eschewed fall detectors because they symbolised frailty and lack of personal agency, with the result that independence was potentially undermined. Personal priorities therefore constitute an important variable to take into account when considering telecare service delivery, particularly in regard to an individual's perceptions of their vulnerability.

Older people in our research agreed that, in order for telecare services to be acceptable and purposeful, they have to be 'tailor-made to that individual'. At the heart of the matter, according to professionals across the focus groups, is the importance of carrying out user-centred assessments that identify need and link this with appropriate provision. Porteus and Brownsell (2000) agree that careful assessment is required so that technology is tailored to the individual, with providers making systems understandable and easy to use by older people and their carers, features that resonate both with Nielsen's (1993) category of usability, mentioned earlier, and also with our participants' views on the question of targeting and scale of provision.

The Department of Heath (2005a) believes that 35 per cent of those living in residential care homes could be supported in ordinary homes or sheltered housing schemes if they had a telecare package to support them. Given that people living in residential care homes tend to be frail and unable to manage many activities of daily living independently, the DH appears to view telecare as potentially targeting older people with high-level care needs. However, according to the background paper on telecare included in the Wanless social care review (King's Fund 2006), there is currently insufficient evidence as regards targeting of telecare services and, as a result, there is debate about whether services should be offered to people with high-level care and support needs or to people generally in order to maximise telecare's preventative role. The Wanless review cites an example of telecare being targeted at people with medium- to high-level care needs as an alternative to residential care but then goes on to state that theoretical cost models support the view that, in the long term, it is those with low- to medium-level care needs who should be targeted if telecare is to result in a reduction in spending on residential care. We should not, however, forget that social services departments, pivotal in providing the support staff and other resources that complete the telecare service, operate strict eligibility criteria that exclude those without the highest care needs (Department of Health 2002c). The Wanless review suggests one way forward, the encouragement of self-funded telecare at an early stage of dependency. A note of caution is necessary here, we believe, because, even if there is a market sufficiently populated by older people interested in purchasing telecare privately, it will remain the responsibility of local social services departments to provide the necessary support systems and, therefore, private telecare purchasers may not be eligible for this back-up if they are deemed to have low-level needs.

The views of older people themselves strongly suggest that telecare should be targeted at those with high-level care needs, individuals who are infirm or ill. Focus group participants repeatedly pointed out that telecare is not relevant if an individual feels capable of managing their condition, and people used phrases such as 'he's a lot older than me', 'he's much more disabled', 'I don't think I class myself as poorly' and 'he really does need something like that' to emphasise a personal reluctance to use telecare services and to direct researchers to those who are more needy in comparison. This reaction to theoretical discussions about telecare may reflect a natural reticence on the part of older people to commit themselves to something new and perhaps only vaguely understood. It is certainly the case that those involved in the pilot project, who had of course agreed to telecare installations and who had high-level care needs because of sight loss and significant health problems, reflected more favourably on the usefulness of telecare. But even these participants were of the opinion that there should not be blanket targeting of telecare at people simply because of their age or their residence in a sheltered housing setting. This point is taken up by the Foundation for Assistive Technology, which argues that the current approach to telecare service development relies on installing large numbers of standardised systems, rather than closely matching telecare to the needs of individuals (Down 2005). A blanket approach to the provision of telecare services potentially undermines independence and choice, but may also exacerbate concerns about confidentiality and surveillance.

Confidentiality and surveillance

A number of informal carers made positive statements about the depth of information that lifestyle monitoring and devices such as wandering alerts can generate, and the likely increased knowledge that carers would subsequently have about a person's risk levels at home. Professionals recognised this benefit and spoke of a consequent better understanding of daily patterns of behaviour, an 'aggregate' picture', suggesting that such data would help build a better understanding of the individual and their routines and potentially lead professionals to worry less about a particular situation.

Across the focus groups, however, there was a general view that telecare-generated data should be subject to strict guidelines of confidentiality, particularly in regard to the potential for commercial companies acquiring lifestyle data and using them to direct marketing strategies or target individuals in order to sell aids or adaptations. Professionals involved in the focus groups were concerned that agencies such as the Department of Social Security (DSS) may obtain access to data about an individual's functioning ability, such as the number of times a person requires attention in the night, and that these data could be used to refute an application for financial benefits such as attendance allowance. These concerns are shared by those examining the private sector's access to medical research databases (Graham & Wood 2003) and government access to citizens' personal information (Whitaker 1999; Lyon 2001). Magnusson and Hanson (2003) indicate that privacy and confidentiality are core issues with ethical implications for telecare service development, because of the risk factors associated with possible uses of personal data and the potential for unjustified paternalism, a concern that Lyon (2001) conceptualises as the care and control motif underlying basic ambiguities of surveillance.

Participants involved in the pilot project initially raised concern that telecare might be an all-seeing, Panopticon-type surveillance system, involving cameras and microphones that log all entries and exits as well as movements in the home. Although interviewees were reassured that this was not the case, they saw a trade-off between close monitoring that safeguarded their welfare and the need to forfeit aspects of privacy as well as relinquish some control over their domestic environment. One participant, for example, found the bed sensor a source of great embarrassment, fearing that it would provide data that informed third parties not only about his occupancy of the bed but also its use by his girlfriend. Pilot project participants also raised an obvious but rather complex related concern, namely that lifestyle monitoring depends on knowing about a person's daily and sometimes hourly lifestyle choices, which could reveal their hoarding of newspapers, cluttering of floor spaces and standards of cleanliness, behaviours that may reflect badly on their lifestyle and management of the home.

According to many participants, we live within a culture of creeping surveillance, a perception that exacerbates the concern already expressed by some older people living in supported housing settings that the existing community alarm systems can feel intrusive, producing a 'sense of being watched', a finding noted in other telecare studies (Brownsell & Bradley 2003; Magnusson & Hanson 2003). For Lyon (2001), the emergence of a surveillance culture reflects society's preoccupation with risk, certainly a central issue in the debate about providing adequate support to vulnerable people.

Risk is a matter intrinsically connected with autonomy and self-determination, not least for many older people who are vulnerable to falls. Brownsell and Hawley (2004) have noted that older people do not always want falls within the home to be known or responded to, for fear of negative consequences such as pressure to relinquish the home and move into institutional care. Additionally, an older person's psychological priorities may differ from those of carers or service providers, a point explored by Ballinger and Payne (2002: 305), who argue that, while service providers are responsible for assessing and minimising physical risk, older people themselves are more concerned with the risk to their identities and 'self-image' when seen as frail or vulnerable. One pilot project participant who had an epilepsy sensor connected to her bed to monitor her heart rate and breathing patterns said that the device made her realise how sensitive she felt about her 'last bit of independence' being stripped away. This participant's feelings personify the contention put forward by Whitaker (1999) that new technologies can reduce the private spheres in which people have traditionally sought refuge and self-definition. Although this interviewee gradually accepted the benefit of this level of intimate monitoring, it was a 'hurdle to get over' on an emotional level. We need, therefore, to be careful about the ways in which telecare services can raise feelings that affect dignity and self-esteem in the home environment.

Behind many of these concerns about the potential for telecare to undermine privacy was the worry that surveillance technology is developing at a rate that could result in human needs being overlooked or ignored. This was most often voiced in the context of participants' anxiety about telecare's potential to replace more traditional and valued forms of hands-on support and care and, in so doing, reduce social inclusion.

Virtual care and social inclusion

Existing forms of support are important to older and disabled people for a number of reasons. Visits from professional carers not only provide the opportunity to monitor a person's well-being at close quarters but also provide a source of interaction with, and information about, the local community and the outside world, helping the housebound person feel socially connected. Furthermore, participants from the caring professions spoke of the potential for routine contacts to identify and highlight subtle changes in a person's condition that telecare devices would not detect. Participants also suggested that such personal contact validates the individual and helps address emotional issues as well as practical tasks.

It is not surprising, perhaps, that older people with basic community alarm systems sometimes use them to engineer human contact that is otherwise missing in their lives. One focus group participant, an alarm call centre manager, spoke of the frequency with which service users press their alarm button, purely to hear a human voice and have 'a chat'. In this way, technology can be used to help foster virtual social contact, but the same manager emphasised the need for more resources to make this a reality. Of course, telecare can enhance virtual care contacts. According to a website providing information about usability and human–computer interaction (Usabilitynews 2007), social inclusion is inherent in the design of 'broadcare' services that provide remote care through video conferencing with carers, friends and family. Participants in our research acknowledged that telecare technology can provide useful virtual contact but emphasised the point that someone who is spending a great deal of time at home, and lives alone, should also have the opportunity to meet people. There was concern that ICT could actually discourage the required effort in this respect, which in turn could adversely affect fitness, mobility and general well-being. In this respect, one informal carer spoke of her husband, a wheelchair user, who uses a computer 'endlessly' but is no longer motivated to have personal contacts.

There is also an argument for regularly maintaining contact with professionals responsible for telecare so that, as personal needs change, the technology is recalibrated to keep pace with change. This was evident in interviews with pilot project participants who reported different routines resulting from changes in medication. It became clear that data from telecare sensors can only be accurately interpreted if there is adequate and up-to-date contextual information about the individual's health and social circumstances, and this is best achieved through regular reassessment and monitoring by professionals.

Nuances in patterns may come about because of changes in medication, or because of a surprise visit by a relative, and so the interpretation of lifestyle monitoring data cannot be a simple process, relying as it does on regular contextual updates.

There is, therefore, a need for a balance between provision of technology and personal contact with carers and support staff, a conclusion reached in a recent study of the acceptability of assistive technology to older people (McCreadie & Tinker 2005). This proper balance may be threatened, however, if telecare is seen as a service that actually replaces hands-on care staff, a fear expressed by members across the groups. Focus group participants could draw on experience of underprovision and cost-cutting in the present health and social care system, leading to the conclusion that telecare may be a convenient way of providing support to vulnerable people while saving money on staff costs. Participants from the caring professions also talked of staffing constraints and a move to implement self-assessment programmes to reduce staff costs. A number of studies have revealed similar concerns about the likelihood of technology leading to increased isolation of service users and decreased interaction with health and social care practitioners (Tang *et al.* 2000; Bowes & McColgan 2002; Hibbert *et al.* 2003). Bowes & McColgan (2003) discovered that those in receipt of smart technology received fewer general practitioner (GP) visits than the 'comparator group' of people who did not have the technology. Such findings reinforce a conclusion reached by Graham and Wood (2003) that digital technology encourages a move away from direct human intervention as surveillance becomes more automated.

The government acknowledges that telecare can 'make a contribution' to meeting potential shortfalls in the social care workforce, but argues that this does not necessarily mean formal carers will no longer be required as they can be deployed to carry out more quality interaction instead of the repeated routine monitoring that telecare devices can provide (Department of Health 2005b). The Audit Commission (2004c) agrees that telecare technologies may usefully replace traditional 'human effort', particularly in situations where staff carry out more mundane tasks. This notion was strongly refuted by participants, for the reasons noted above. However, the government also offers words of caution in respect of potential replacement of carers when it claims that society must not permit 'new technologies to control or isolate us ... [as] human contact is vital to maintaining quality of life' and that innovations such as telecare must therefore complement traditional forms of care, not replace them (Department of Health 2005a: 5). Our research suggests that, if telecare is to be seen in terms of its potential to complement and integrate forms of care service delivery, there are a number of organisational and resource issues that need addressing.

Integration and resourcing of telecare and complementary services

Participants across the focus groups as well as those included in the pilot project were keen to tell us that in their view telecare should be provided as part of a community care package, rather than as a stand-alone service. One reason for this was that such integration would take proper account of older people's social inclusion and the importance to them of human support, an issue we have discussed. Another reason put forward with some strength is that telecare will necessitate a rigorous, well-resourced and collaborative professional approach to have credibility as a service. This perception is shared by government and relevant agencies. The Warner review (King's Fund 2006: 2) claims that telecare developments will 'combine [telecare] with case management, disease management, self-care and integrated teams'. Warner further argues that telecare should be part of a 'whole systems' approach, improving quality of care as an adjunct to and not a replacement of home care services. By way of example, Warner refers to a rural virtual care model, which is attempting to link telecare with the commissioning and delivery of domiciliary care and extra care housing for older people. Across government departments and public and private sector agencies, there is common cause for the integration of telecare with health, housing and social care services (Department of Health 2005a; SSIA 2007; TSA 2007).

There is, then, no shortage of supporters for the cause of integration. But as our research participants point out, telecare and its integration with allied services cannot move forward unless there is adequate organisation and resourcing of support systems. In this respect, some participants raised doubts about whether services are sufficiently resourced to provide an ongoing telecare service, 24 hours each day, given their experience of local reductions in social services budgets and agencies struggling to cope with needs, whether it be for domiciliary care or for aids and adaptations. And participants were very clear that telecare would require a 24-hour back-up service of professional carers, not a service that relies on informal carers to shoulder the burden. The government has stated that telecare can relieve some of the burdens and pressures experienced by informal carers, for reasons stated earlier when discussing telecare's ability to provide close monitoring of an individual's behaviour and activities. However, informal carers are also likely to be the first point of contact when a telecare device raises an alert and, in our focus groups, participants who provide informal care voiced concern that their involvement would be seen as a cheap alternative to statutory services and that telecare could result in more demands being made on informal carers. As one carer commented in a focus group, if the policy behind telecare is to keep people at home longer, informal care is likely to be exploited by agencies trying to save money. Those professionals involved in the focus groups expressed sympathy with such sentiments and confirmed that a great deal of care in the community currently depends on informal care.

Professionals also agreed with the view that support and care services are often stretched, and some gave examples of instances in which older people are not supported sufficiently in the community at the present time. Participants were aware of the challenge presented by telecare in terms of its 24-hour remit and stated that the volume of alerts triggered by telecare devices could become significant if telecare is rolled out into the mainstream, necessitating a sufficiently robust and flexible system of support that can respond appropriately. Some professionals indicated that a reconfiguration or remodelling of services may be required, a conclusion also reached by technology specialists researching in this field, who argue that technology as a support tool is only as effective as the speedy availability of appropriate professional care services (Lyall 2005). Additionally, a speedy response would have to be provided by at least two staff responding to an alert in cases of falls, and such staff would also have to be trained so they could respond to the needs of people with sensory and cognitive impairments. Collaboration may therefore be very important, and alarm call centres are likely to be pivotal in coordinating a unified service response. However, according to the experience of one of our participants, the manager of an alarm centre, his privatised service has fewer links than he would like with statutory agencies. Some commentators worry that privatised, centralised call centres will become commonplace as the telecare client base grows and as local authorities experience increasing pressure to reduce costs, with the consequent loss of local response and the dilution of specialist services (Down 2005).

Some of these resource issues are implicitly acknowledged in the Warner review (King's Fund 2006), which states that the integration of telecare development with complementary services is not a straightforward proposition, as integration raises a number of administrative and financial questions, and that telecare has important implications for the deployment of staff. Warner goes on to say that there need to be new methods of working as part of a 'whole systems approach', a concept not described in detail. Recent projects cited in the Warner review suggest that workload will increase as a result of telecare, with one project estimating a threefold increase in the workload of the appointed careline provider, due to both the complexity of the equipment and the high volume of calls. Additionally, telecare implementation has to take account of organisational constraints and administrative challenges inherent in partnership operations (Barlow *et al*. 2005). Indeed, the Warner review concludes that the biggest challenges in terms of mainstreaming telecare will be creating the required organisational structures, retraining staff and deciding how to apportion costs.

Conclusions

This chapter began with an account of focus group participants' views about telecare technology, views that led some to think creatively about possible applications of the technology to their own personal situations and suggest innovative developments of the technology. This strongly indicates that older people and their carers are prepared to look favourably at new supportive technologies and embrace the potential offered by telecare. Potential users and pilot project participants involved in our research have also raised concerns and questions that providers need to understand and resolve if public endorsement of telecare is to be maintained. In this respect, the importance of older people's values and beliefs, relevant to Nielsen's concept of social acceptability, should not be underestimated, reflecting as they do deeply held convictions about maintaining privacy, autonomy and self-determination. Providers and policy-makers also have to grapple with the gauntlet thrown down by Wanless, that in order for telecare to be an effective and economical source of support, it has to be collaboratively integrated with other forms of community care and properly resourced. Professional staff constitute the most expensive aspect of a telecare service, a fact that tends to be obscured in the heat of discussions about new technological advances. Our research makes clear that, without adequate staff resources and back-up services, telecare technology is likely to be ineffective and will not command the interest or commitment of potential users. We therefore believe that the issues raised in our research merit serious consideration, if government money earmarked for preventative technology is to be well spent and telecare's potential role in an ageing society is to be fully realised.

Notes

1 The research was carried out under EPSRC's EQUAL Programme (grant number GR/S 29058/01). The consortium includes Imperial College London, University College London, Dundee University, Barnsley District General Hospital NHS Trust, Anchor Trust, Thomas Pocklington Trust and Tunstall Telecom Ltd.

5 Information and communications technologies and health care

User-centred devices and patient work

Andrew Webster

Introduction: ubiquitous computing

> The design and implementation of new ICTs should be seen as an iterative process where the users are central. Experimentation and evaluation are also key components. ICTs should be designed with close involvement from users and around the ways in which people work. This involves having clearly identified objectives to ensure that the technologies can solve specific healthcare problems, not assuming any existing technologies designed originally for non-healthcare solutions will work.
>
> Royal Society (2006)

This quotation is taken from a recently completed analysis by the Royal Society of the role of information and communication technologies (ICTs) within the UK health care system today. It emphasises the role the user plays – or should play – in the design and purpose of such technologies, especially where these are to be deployed outside the conventional clinical context of the hospital or other clinical sites. Most importantly, it suggests that difficulties can arise when these systems are principally designed to be used in clinical settings but used elsewhere, failing to recognise the actual context of use. This chapter examines the particular problems that can arise when the responsibility for using e-health technology falls on older patients enrolled as active agents in managing their own diagnosis and treatment through the use of ICTs in non-clinical settings. This delegation of responsibility to the older user/patient is characteristic of health care today, not just in e-health, but also more widely as part of a discourse of a patient-centred and so patient 'empowered' engagement with medicine. However, while there are positive benefits to be derived from inviting older people to play a greater role in managing their condition outside the clinic, the experience that patients have of this process and the unintended effects it can generate raise complex unforeseen difficulties for them as end-users.

These difficulties are in part a reflection of what Urry (2000: 18) has called the 'contingent ordering' of contemporary social life resulting precisely from the attempt to tie down and order social relations, technologies and their use and meaning. The latter is evident for example in the time and effort devoted to the evaluation and assessment of health interventions (such as drugs, devices and therapies) within 'evidence-based' medicine. The former is just as evident when such evaluations are actually made and used to inform decisions, for it is then that contingency and the mess of practice loom large (May *et al.* 2005). Research on the play of ICT systems within specific sociotechnical settings – such as hospitals – reveals both these dynamics at work (Berg & Goorman 1999; Timmermans & Berg 2003).

Beneath the polished presence of the device, the machine, ICT systems are embedded, invisibly, within the physical and virtual environment, as so-called 'ubiquitous computing' deploying 'ambient intelligence' (Ducatel 2000; Woolgar 2002). Space becomes digitally framed and tracked, as we see in the growth of radio frequency identity tags (RFID) that monitor and report the movements of objects in space and time (Crang & Graham 2007). Within the contexts of clinical practice, e-health systems now allow for the deployment of devices that are embedded as biosensors within patients' bodies, devices that convert a biological response into a digital electrical signal to be tracked remotely and logged by a central server monitoring a person's condition, such as their blood pressure. Commercial organisations provide digital scanning services that allow an individual to provide regular reports on their 'body mass index' to determine whether they are dieting effectively. As Virilio (1998: 53) has observed, we 'have to cope with technology inhabiting us. "Smart pills" are developed which are able to transmit information on nerve functions or blood flows to distant monitoring facilities'. Virilio's dystopic view is that eventually people will effectively function as 'citizen-terminals' where we are 'decked out to the eyeballs with interactive prostheses' (ibid.: 20). This might seem somewhat exaggerated but, on the contrary, health care ICT developers are now speaking of the 'pervasive' patient-based communications that will function precisely in this way using body sensors embedded in clothing. It is even conceivable that such sensors could be networked across families whose members have a specific (inherited) disorder to track and map the onset of familial disease or other abnormalities. E-health is also found within buildings, such as 'smart homes' for older people or the chronically ill, including the monitoring and remote imaging systems used in telecare and telemedicine (Barlow *et al.* 2006).

Digital information is highly mobile and also, as a result, potentially insecure as it moves across networks and interoperable processing systems. This capacity for the classification and mobilisation of large data sets has been exploited by some of the major institutions in society, including those within the health care system. The mix of digital technologies in the e-health domain is increasingly being used to perform or assist in the clinical performance of the diagnosis, monitoring and management of patients. Indeed, this has been seen as a shift from the management of places in conventional institutional settings (such as the hospital) to management through 'extitutional technologies' that control through programme, tracking and feedback (Domènech *et al.* 2006). The UK's National Health Service (NHS) is investing up to £20 billion in the

Connecting for Health ICT system that will, in theory, allow for the seamless movement of information on patients across relevant health care practitioners. In practice, the system has been far from stable and its utility far from self-evident to the multiplicity of local and regional trusts that populate the NHS. Beyond its clinical use, e-health serves a broader organisational and bureaucratic purpose to allow the auditing, standardisation and surveillance of practice and its resource needs and demands. As I have argued elsewhere (Webster 2002, 2007), the contemporary medical world is becoming increasingly 'informaticised'.

These developments, as with any disruptive technology, generate not only new types of social relationships – with our bodies, our kin, as well as between medics, to the state – but also new risks and threats. For example, telehealth care can be said to have contradictory effects: on the one hand, it is deployed in order to enhance older patients' autonomy (by allowing them to remain at home, for example); on the other hand, for it to work, patients must be compliant to be remotely 'activated' through a distributed information system infrastructure (Mort *et al.* 2003). Patient carers are caught up in this process at the same time and required to carry an ever increasing burden of responsibility for health. Moreover, the volume and flow of information creates new risks with regard to an individual's rights to privacy and concerns over who has authorised access to patient information.

It is important to ask whether these developments have particular implications for patients and especially older patients. I go on to examine these in more detail below, but it is worth noting that it would be unwise to assume that ICT systems affect 'patients-as-such' in a uniform way, whatever their age. Within the UK, for example, the diffusion and take-up of new ICT systems is geographically highly uneven, involves a diverse array of products that may be more, or less, interoperable and difficult to coordinate, and a variety of commercial providers with different definitions of patient need and models of the context of use. Patients' experience of e-health is likely therefore to be equally diverse and of more, or less, personal utility and value. Information 'flows' will thereby be mediated by the uneven topography of the e-healthscape and will in turn be subject to various translations along the way (Latour 2005; Wathen *et al.* 2008).

The turn to patient-centredness

While it might have been presumed that health care systems serve patient interests and to that extent put the patient at the centre of health care, what this has typically meant is that the patient acts as an object of medical intervention subject to the clinical gaze (Foucault 1975), effectively a 'doctor-centred' rather than patient-centred model (May *et al.* 2004). The patient here is configured to play the 'sick role' (Parsons 1951) carrying certain rights and obligations that must be performed in order to secure both medical and carer support and to provide a socially legitimate route from ill-health to recovery.

While this configuring of the patient still prevails, it obtains primarily to those suffering from acute and so remediable sickness. The growth of chronic illnesses associated with an ageing society means that most older patients who engage with the health care system cannot be managed in this way, posing both clinical and parallel resource demands. It is then not surprising to see the turn to patient-centred medicine for this redefines the boundaries of responsibility for care, while at the same time delegating some of the resource needs it has direct to the patients and carers themselves.

There are a number of discursive shifts – especially in policy arenas – associated with this process. One invokes the move from the passive patient to an active patient, who is a participant in the care process. This is illustrated by the *Expert Patient Programme* initiated by the UK government in 2001 that is designed to enhance self-management and, in the long term, generate public health and financial gains (Lorig 2002). Evidence relating to the actual efficacy of this programme on patient outcomes is thin and fails to take account of the normal process through which improvement occurs within many patients over time, the 'duration effects' (see Taylor & Bury 2007). A second sense in which patient-centredness has become part of a wider discursive repertoire relates to the rapid and extensive growth of the collective patient as embodied in patient advocacy groups and patient charities: here, the experience and needs of the individual patient as a user of medicine are mobilised through formal patient organisations. This is often couched in a language not only of need but rights over health resources, a move from being merely a sick patient to a highly politicised patient-citizen. Sometimes, this involves a set of demands to access new medicines – for experimental drugs say – and sometimes to resist medical interventions driven by public health regimes, as in the case of anti-vaccination groups (Hobson-West 2007).

It is, though, the embrace in broader terms of the notion of 'patient-centred medicine' by most health care systems that marks out and informs many of the developments in contemporary health care delivery, including those related to the use of ICT-dependent devices. Apart from specific initiatives such as the *Expert Patient Programme* noted above, there are a number of other aspects to this, not always working in the same direction. For example, patient-centredness is driven by the state's attempt to reduce the burden it carries of hospital care: not only does this put more responsibilities on general practitioners' clinics to offer a wider range of specialist services (such as minor operations), it also seeks to relocate some health care delivery to the home setting, or the wider community, where appropriate. This can reduce the costs of care and, as some evidence suggests (Wolpert & Anderson 2001), provide clinical benefit for patients. On the other hand, patient-centredness invokes the language of patient 'choice' and the adoption of policies that allow patients to choose which hospital they might prefer to attend. This could have the effect of increasing the costs, at least administratively, for the hospital sector, and does in turn depend on robust ICT systems to provide information about what is actually available.

Either aspect places more responsibility on the shoulders of patients to manage their illness. As Lupton (1996) has argued, we cannot assume that patients welcome this and will at times be much more likely to prefer that practitioners take primary responsibility for their health care. Indeed, if one considers the extensive body of work on patient narratives in managing chronic illness (see e.g. Kleinman 1988; Hyden 1997; Bury 2001; Faircloth *et al.* 2004), it is clear that patients have changing needs over time, with more or less dependency on formal medical care. This means that the 'centre' of care may well move as circumstances change, as patients make sense of their illness within the wider biography of the self. Such narratives are at least as much (if not more likely to be) affective rather than cognitive in their framing, reflecting the changing circumstances of the patient and the levels of anxiety they may raise.

This argument suggests that the use of ICT systems as part of a push towards patient-centred medicine, especially in home-based contexts, may both empower older patients but also increase existing or create new anxieties. In order to see how this can occur, I turn now to a detailed analysis of the use of remote monitoring of older patients' cardiac problems through the use of electrocardiograms (ECG) in the home, linked to a clinical centre through the telephone. The account draws on Oudshoorn (2008) who examined the ways in which patients used and made sense of this telemonitoring device designed to check and report on irregular heart rhythms.

Invisible work and distributed responsibilities

Before elaborating on Oudshoorn's work, it is important to make two general points about user–technology relations, both drawn from science and technology studies (STS). The first is that there is a recursive effect between technology and user, each co-constructing the other. That is, the meaning and utility of technologies are not pre-inscribed as essential properties but created through and in their context of use. So for example, as Saetnan (2002) has shown, the value and meaning of closed circuit television (CCTV) surveillance is variously constructed as 'protective, invasive, acceptable here, not acceptable there' and so on. This has implications for the attempt by technology designers who endeavour to configure or materialise their prospective user within the product itself – a strategy that is likely to fail (McLaughlin *et al.* 1999; Oudshoorn & Pinch 2003). The second point is that, while this process of co-construction draws attention to the (inter)active, very visible engagement of user and technology, other work has pointed to the ways in which this co-construction is not completely open or rendered in visible ways (Mort *et al.* 2008). Technology even as co-constructed often closes down options and choices, and may well do so in a much less visible way (Bowker & Star 1999). This is especially true of ICT systems and the infrastructural networks through which they are made to function, for these enable, or as Star (1999) says, encode some possibilities for action and exclude others.

These two themes – of the plasticity and the constraints of socio-technology – shape how co-construction is enacted in particular spaces and times, and is of relevance to Oudshoorn's analysis of the home-based ECG. As we shall see, the system is only made to function through active investment by the patient while at the same time delimiting how such an investment can be made. This investment is, according to Oudshoorn, a form of 'work' that, while clearly visible and evident to both the user and the analyst-ethnographer, goes unrecognised by the system designers.

Oudshoorn explores first the ways in which technologies are only made workable through the participation of a network of actors (and in Latour's (1987) terms, actants); it is precisely the articulation of their work that makes technologies workable. This is especially so in regard to telemedicine, which 'works' through the combined agency of device(s), patients, clinicians, IT engineers and manu-facturers, as well as at a wider level, the telecommunications platform upon which the whole system depends (such as broadband, satellite technology and so on). Crucial to her argument is the work that patients have to undertake, for this involves their acting as 'diagnostic agents'. People have routinely self-diagnosed, of course, as Kleinman (1988) argued many years ago, within what he called the 'cultural health system'. In the case of the ECG study, however, the diagnostics are undertaken as part of the *clinical* health system, so is markedly different. Before we discuss this, some further details of Oudshoorn's study are in order.

Oudshoorn contacted ninety-five patients in the Netherlands (in 2004/5) who numbered among a larger group who had agreed to be wired up with an ECG attached to their bodies as part of a telemedical trial in remote monitoring of chronic heart arrhythmia. With one or two exceptions, the majority of the respondents were older patients. The ECG recorder is strapped to the waist with electrodes attached to the wall of the chest. The patients must then press a record button and, after four occasions of doing so, must then download the recording through a telephone call made to the telemedical centre. They do this by holding up the device to the phone speaker and waiting until they hear a 'beep' sound indicating it has been received; they then delete the recordings and ensure all the wiring and contacts are still in place and not damaged in any way.

This seems relatively straightforward, and we can assume that the designers of this system had a similar attitude towards its simplicity and value to that expressed in an equivalent monitoring system deployed in Sweden (see Box 5.1).

As Oudshoorn's study shows, however, this version of events seriously understates the invisible work that patients and indeed the other actors involved – the nurses and physicians – have to undertake to make the system work. The key point the study makes though is that tasks once conducted by practitioners are now delegated to patients. What are these tasks?

There are two forms of work the patient must undertake. First, there are instrumental tasks, that is to say those tasks that depend on observing certain practical procedures such as checking the functioning and condition of the wiring. This is a form of work that is quite visible and requires following explicit instructions provided by the telemedical centre. The more invisible work

Box 5.1 The Promise of Telemonitoring

With the Home Diagnosis and Monitoring Set, patients suffering from chronic heart failure can easily make a daily check of parameters that give important indications of their health. Electrodes on the sensor unit, carried in the vest, monitor the selected biological parameters. These are transferred wirelessly to the home unit for analysis and storage, and then sent on to a hospital or care centre. This provides a better diagnostic basis for treatment and reduces the number of readmissions.

UMEA Institute of Design (2006)

relates to patients taking on the role of 'diagnostic agents'. The following captures its central challenge for the patient:

In the new 'geography of responsibilities' introduced by the ambulatory ECG recorder, the most difficult task is delegated to patients: they are expected to catch the right moment to register an ECG that shows their heart rate dysfunction. Many patients experienced it as difficult to decide which moment they should choose to register an ECG.

Oudshoorn (2008: 276)

Deciding the right moment to make the recording was not something that the patients had any clear guidance about, especially in respect to what was to be regarded as serious enough to warrant pressing the record button on the ECG. Patients understood their heart problems within and through the experiences of their everyday lives: some for example were used to more frequent arrhythmia during the night so did not feel it appropriate to press the button then. Others experienced heart palpitations in very short bursts that might or might not be properly captured by the ECG, while still others had a sense that their heart might go into arrhythmia solely as a result of *other* conditions, or co-morbidities, that they had. As one said (ibid.: 277):

Sometimes I was tired but did not know whether it was caused by my heart. I can be tired because I am short of breath as well

woman, aged 81

And indeed, as Oudshoorn observes, precisely because many of the respondents were in poor health, they were less likely to be able to use the ECG with any confidence or degree of control. As one said (ibid.: 277):

Sometimes I felt very weak and almost fainted. At such moments you don't think of the recorder at all. When it was over I thought that pushing the button did not make sense any more

woman, aged 84

In addition, the wearing of the recorder could create its own anxieties and trigger the very palpitations it was supposed to capture. In short, patients had to 'read' their bodies and come to a judgement, and so decision, about whether to trigger the ECG.

Once recordings has been taken, patients were also then required to use their telephones in a way that did not inspire confidence in the technological system: they found it difficult to accept that holding the ECG device to the telephone speaker would send a message down the line to the centre. In some cases, patients only came to accept that this was possible when they had sight of the paper printout from their despatch at a later date. Moreover, as telephones varied (the size of the mouthpiece for example), there were no standardised instructions about how far from or near to the handset the ECG should be, as Oudshoorn argues:

> ... patients had to figure out the optimal distance between the recorder and the phone on their own. The articulation work of patients thus also consisted of learning new skills to co-ordinate the use of two technological devices and to build trust in the new technology.

Oudshoorn goes on to describe the other hidden tasks that the other actors in the telemonitoring system had to undertake to ensure it became workable, much of which involved reassuring patients that, despite their distance from the doctors and nurses, they were being looked after effectively, and we might add, affectively. As is remarked:

> Although affective work is an important aspect of healthcare in general, it seems to be more imperative in healthcare at a distance.
>
> Oudshoorn (2008: 283)

Going beyond Oudshoorn's analysis, it is also as important to stress the way in which this diagnostic work was being done in the *home*. We noted earlier that the translation of diagnostic devices from a clinical to a domestic setting is fraught with problems. The 'domestication' (Silverstone & Hirsch 1992; Lie & Sørensen 1996) of technologies by the user/consumer is a term that has been used to describe the ways in which technologies are appropriated, 'tamed' and exploited by the consumer to their own ends. In the case of the ECG, the domestication process is only partly apparent inasmuch as it centres on managing the technology in a domestic setting but, beyond that, there is little sense of a confident and competent taming of the system by the patient. Patients had to develop a series of strategies to bring the system under their sense of control – such as triggering heart palpitations directly by walking up and down stairs vigorously – strategies that from a clinical perspective might have been regarded as far from desirable. Domestication would instead require that objects are incorporated into people's daily routines, rather than only through a disruption of them; indeed, it could be argued that, in order to manage the arrhythmia of the heart, the ECG users had to create an arrhythmia of their daily lives.

This disruptive process has been seen in research elsewhere (Heaton *et al*. 2005) reporting on the use of hospital-derived machines and devices for 'technology-dependent' children, those who may require ventilators, feeding tubes, dialysis and so on not merely to keep going but to stay alive. Heaton *et al*. (2005) found that households' normal social rhythms were often incompatible with the regimes that were required to be followed by parents, other carers and siblings.

Moreover, just as Oudshoorn identified the diagnostic tasks that older patients had to perform, so similar clinically related tasks (what they call 'technical care') were taken on by the parents of these children. These were quite extensive:

> Technical care involved a range of activities, namely: assisting the child when she or he was using a device; monitoring the child by close visual observation and/or use of secondary devices; managing the equipment (e.g. cleaning and preparing it for use, ordering supplies, and managing stocks); maintaining the interface between the device and the body [e.g. care of entry and exit sites (re)placement of tubes]; accessing technical support from service providers (including hospitals, community services, companies who supply equipment and consumables); and providing technical support to others through training formal or informal carers.
>
> Heaton *et al*. (2005: 446)

In Heaton *et al*. (2005), then, we see similar dynamics at work to those identified by Oudshoorn, this time for those experiencing poor health at the other end of the life course and, again, an emphasis is placed on the need to understand both the tasks and the specific (home-based) settings in which these were performed, and crucially *when* they were so. The e-health component is clearly less significant (although not entirely absent) in Heaton's study, but its value is in demonstrating the broad range of tasks that are delegated to intermediary carers (here primarily the children's parents), a range, although varying in form and content, that we might expect to see as telemedicine applications in home-based settings grow and become more prevalent for a variety of conditions among older patients. Both diagnostic and 'technical care' will require work by both patient and carer, and it is likely to be highly invisible to system designers.

Discussion: managing digital uncertainties

Innovative developments in the field of e-health, as in many other areas of contemporary science such as stem cell research (Webster & Eriksson 2008), carry both greater power and higher levels of risk and provisionality that can only be managed through *distributing* responsibility for them across a wide range of social, economic and political actors and networks within and beyond the clinic. One way of seeing this is through reference to MacKenzie's (1998) analysis of what he called the 'certainty trough', a concept he developed during his research on something very far removed from e-health – missile guidance systems – but which has some utility here. MacKenzie argued that those technical experts most close to innovative technologies are aware of their contingencies and uncertainties (but keep this within their local networks), while those more distant (in the middle of the curve) with less technical understanding of a field have to depend and trust on others' (such as government, professionals, etc.) representations of it. At the right-hand side of the curve are those who have serious reservations about the field because they have an understanding of the risks and dangers it poses, and indeed may be quite hostile to its development. Nuclear power might be a good illustration of this. Together, these different positions produce the trough of certainty shown in Figure 5.1.

Curve A relates to MacKenzie's argument that there is an inverse relationship between the level of uncertainty about a field of science and technology and the relative proximity in which its principal knowledge claims are produced. Curve A is based on MacKenzie's original concept with those in the top left-hand area of the curve most committed (despite uncertainties), those at the extreme right of the curve most alienated (because of uncertainties) and those in the middle of the 'trough' such as policy-makers and/or users who embrace the new sociotechnology – here e-health – more certain of its merits and putative utility, where the technology is black-boxed such that no detailed understanding of its inner working is required.

Much of science and technology can be characterised in this way. Indeed, we need not assume that those occupying a position low in the trough of certainty

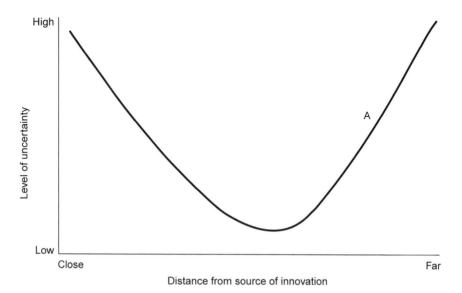

Figure 5.1 The trough of certainty

need be outside of science. Evidence suggests that, in many areas of contemporary science and technology, such as proteomics, scientists acquire highly sophisticated black-boxed technologies from vendors to help automate the production of large-scale data sets, without necessarily understanding in full how the equipment (such as late-generation microarrays) works in detail, so-called 'kit-science'. This can of course lead to a huge increase in data and a situation in which the ability to create data exceeds the ability to use it effectively.

Curve B in Figure 5.2 suggests how Mackenzie's model might apply across a broad range of social actors within and outside technological innovation, redrawn to show how a greater number of social actors are involved in acknowledging and taking responsibility for the provisionality of the innovation, here telemonitoring. This flattening of the curve as the distribution of uncertainties is delegated to a greater number of actors may well become increasingly common across the health devices and technologies as they become more technically complex and deployed in non-clinical ('extitutional') settings. On the one hand, black-boxing still occurs either as standards or as standardised equipment and protocols that the patient/user and/or intermediary carers must follow but, on the other, with a greater obligation passed to the user to understand and work with the contingencies embedded in the system.

Conclusion

Technological developments that allow individuals to monitor and treat themselves will result in considerable changes to the current health care delivery system in the next 10–15 years. Unlike the conventional sick role, where

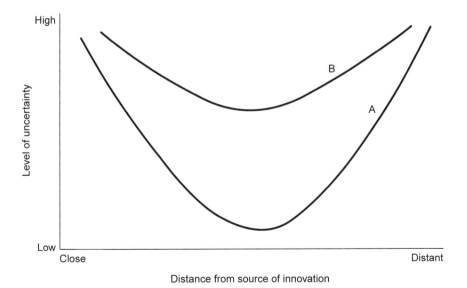

Figure 5.2 The delegation and repositioning of uncertainty to users

there are various rights and responsibilities that patients and those around them enjoy and must observe, the e-health 'sick role' is rather different in its performance, requiring the patient to diagnose and give an account of their illness not merely at a distance but also through determining the boundaries between normal and abnormal readings. This is clearly patient-centred both spatially and diagnostically, raising questions about the extra burden of responsibility placed on patients, who have to manage with uncertainties that have conventionally been resolved by the physician. The work that patients/users must do to deal with the uncertainties they face is rarely acknowledged within telehealth care systems and their design, as we saw above in the extract that appears in Box 5.1. The delegation of uncertainty shown in Figure 5.2 may well increase risks to patient safety, in part by encouraging inappropriate coping mechanisms (such as trying to trigger a palpitation to generate a reading for the telecentre). Indeed, as the Royal Society report, with which this chapter opened, noted, precisely because of the new responsibilities and risks faced by older patients, it may well be the case that there will a large proportion of older people in the UK (and elsewhere) who will have little or no desire to 'empower' themselves. Even those patients who are more willing and who are prescribed such systems may use them selectively and fail the compliance model upon which they depend for their utility. Those who are also deemed not to meet the requirements of the system could become further marginalised from health care if non-digital routes are reduced as a result of telemedicine. Intermediary carers are being asked to shoulder some of the responsibility, but we need to ask how far the social relationships within the family household can act as the medium through which new responsibilities can be taken up. It was clear from Heaton's study that existing familial capacities for managing chronic care are limited and depend on prolonged and extensive efforts by some members of the family to make things work.

The advent of home-based e-health also raises wider questions about clinical governance in telemedicine. The delegation of responsibility to the patient with respect to their health is built into the system's design but with limited or no information about how best to go about this. In order to make it work, patients in Oudshoorn's study had to become competent diagnostic agents, which took not only time but the learning of new skills and new forms of 'articulation' with other actors within the system. Much then depends on how these others respond to the anxieties that the system creates and how they relate to each other in monitoring patient needs at a distance. It also depends on a wider policy and resource-related question as to who is responsible for maintaining the system.

The uncertainties that were once managed and to some extent hidden in conventional doctor–patient relations surface and are more directly experienced by the patient (such as defining normality). Telehealth care for older patients needs to be designed in such a way as to ensure that the additional responsibilities that patients face have the institutional back-up when and where needed and do not depend exclusively on extitutional processes. The design and implementation of new telemedical systems should be seen as an iterative process between designer and user (captured by Suchman's (2002) term 'design in use') especially in terms of understanding what is to be monitored and why – the social ontology of the informatics system – and what decision rules and guidance are to be built in. As Mort *et al.* (2008) have argued recently:

> [E]xperiential knowledge co-produced by the patient and the clinician could influence the design, practice, and evaluation of the system. The possibility of co-construction, for example, taking knowledge generated in the clinic back into the domains of evidence and design, draws an important link between technology as innovation and technology as governance.

Apart from securing better design and accountability, such an approach is more likely to acknowledge the actual redistribution of uncertainties and risks that characterise the ways in which innovation systems operate in the contemporary era, as suggested in Figure 5.2. This embrace of uncertainty may also help to dampen down expectations about the 'promise' that a field holds (Borup *et al.* 2006) and help to foster a more precautionary approach to its long-term adoption and so a more effective, transparent form of governance in e-health, which will be important for patients and carers wherever they are located on the life course.

6 Networked carers

Digital exclusion or digital empowerment?[1]

John Powell

Abstract

Given the current ageing population, by 2025, there will be over 1 million people with dementia in the UK. Large numbers of people provide informal care to people with dementia. The economic, social and psychological needs of carers of people with dementia can be huge. The networked society offers theoretical benefits to these carers, but also potential threats. In this chapter, these issues are examined with reference to previous studies of networked interventions to support carers of people with dementia. Information and communication technologies (ICTs) can support the expert carer to become informed, engage with others and organise socially and politically; the removal of traditional access barriers can reduce the isolation of carers through facilitating interaction with peers for social support, and with health, social and commercial organisations for the remote delivery of services; remote monitoring can allow caring at a distance and can provide visual and geographical monitoring as well as being linked to assistive devices and smart home technology. However, problems can be created through such issues as digital exclusion, digital abuse, depersonalisation and threats to privacy.

Introduction

Four major issues facing health and social care policy-makers at the start of the twenty-first century are the management of long-term chronic conditions, the ageing population and the implications this will have for age-related disease prevalence, the rise of the informed, empowered consumer and the development of new e-health technologies. Demographic change and improvements in disease management mean that not only will more people live longer with chronic illnesses, but there will also be fewer younger family carers and fewer active workers contributing to the UK welfare state through taxation. Health and social care systems faced with an inevitable and potentially unsustainable rise in care costs are now putting much emphasis on the development of self-care knowledge and skills among 'expert patients' and the promotion of home disease management. ICTs are widely seen as providing the tools to enable this shift from the hospital to the home, from the professionals to the patients. In the UK, the economic benefits of such an approach have been explicitly recorded in reports prepared for the UK Treasury by Sir Derek Wanless (Wanless 2002, 2004). These reports described a 'fully engaged' scenario of empowered patients becoming involved in their care, supported by technology. At the same time, both carers and older people with mental health problems are a current priority for the National Health Service (NHS). In this chapter, I will examine the potential role that new ICTs can play in supporting carers of people with dementia and discuss the barriers and facilitators to such technologies.

Background

Dementia is a condition of progressive global impairment of higher cortical functions associated with underlying brain disease. There is a decline in both memory and thinking which is sufficient to impair personal activities of daily living. Dementia affects at least 5 per cent of people over age 65 and 20 per cent of people over age 80 (Melzer *et al.* 1994). It is estimated that dementia affects 24.3 million people worldwide, with 4 to 6 million new cases each year (Ferri *et al.* 2005). The Alzheimer's Society estimates there are currently over 700,000 people with dementia in the UK and, given the ageing population, this is expected to rise to over 1 million by 2025 (Knapp & Prince 2007).

The majority of dementia sufferers are cared for at home (Arksey *et al.* 2004). Carers tend to be women and tend to be the spouse or child of the person with dementia. The economic, social and psychological burden on carers is huge, and their practical needs for support, as well as their needs in relation to the emotional impact of caring, are especially high (Arksey *et al.* 2004). It is well established that family carers often suffer from social isolation as well as having significant needs for information (Levin 1997). It is also clear that psychological morbidity, including serious depression, is very common among carers of people with dementia (Coope *et al.* 1995; Livingstone *et al.* 1996). Psychosocial support has been shown to be of some benefit to these carers (Cooke *et al.* 2001; Pusey & Richards 2001). Carers' social networks also play important roles in the caring career (Cohen *et al.* 1994; McGarry & Arthur 2001).

Technologies are increasingly being used to provide support to people with dementia and their carers and to prolong community living. Previous work in this area has mainly involved assistive devices – fairly simple electronic gadgets such as movement sensors that assist with a particular activity of daily living. Such technologies come under the banner of 'telecare', which also describes more sophisticated systems of devices, seen in 'smart homes', and increasingly complex intelligent surveillance systems which can (for example) identify unusual patterns of behaviour.

In the UK, the last few years have seen enormous investment in telecare at a national and local level. Currently, there are three centrally funded major

demonstrator projects in progress to further investigate the benefits and possibilities. The dominant discourse is one of telecare being a key part of the
solution to demographic change and shifting the management of long-term
chronic conditions from the professional to the patient, and from the hospital
to the home. At the same time, such interventions can also move responsibilities and risks from the state to the individual. Of course, prolonged community living may not be the goal for all carers, and Askham (1998) has
defined 'carer support' as any intervention that assists a carer in deciding
whether to take up, continue or terminate the caring role (Askham 1998).
Nevertheless, the discourse of telecare is one of maintaining and prolonging
home-based assistance.

New networked ICTs such as the Internet and related technologies are now
emerging as tools to help carers reduce isolation, seek health information and
support, undertake remote consultations, share experiences with others, organise
in virtual communities and undertake other activities that ease the burden of
caring which may not be directly related to health or social care, for example
Internet shopping. Such benefits may possibly lead to improvements in quality
of life for carers and avoid or delay unwanted transfer of the person they are
caring for to an institutional setting. Convergence of digital technologies will
mean that while, in this chapter, I will often refer to the Internet as a shorthand,
in future, the same technologies will be available through multiple platforms
such as interactive digital television and mobile telephones.

Many carers of people with dementia are spouse carers and therefore belong
to a generation that tends to be less familiar with tools such as the Internet.
This is changing, partly as existing members of this generation increase their
use of new ICTs and mainly due to a cohort effect as the more computer-literate
generations age. In the UK in 2007, 59 per cent of 55–64 year olds used the
Internet in the preceding 3 months, and 24 per cent of those aged 65 or over
had done so. The figures for 2006 were 52 per cent and 15 per cent. In 2003, a
survey of clients at a UK memory clinic where people with suspected dementia
are assessed showed that, although at that time only 27 per cent of patients
and carers had used the Internet as an information source, 82 per cent would
access websites suggested by clinic staff (Larner 2003).

Potential benefits and threats of networked technologies

Castells (2000) has described the recent emergence of the network society as a
new variant of capitalism, where networks are the dominant social structure.
Castells sees the transformation of society as being, in part, driven by technological innovation, although his thesis is not one of technological determinism.
Information and information technology are central to a restructured capitalism where industry is less labour intensive and the means of production are
characterised by flexibility and geographical dispersion, although integrated at
a global level. In this network society, there is a shift in power from the state
to the producers of culture. Castells sees a breakdown of the identities of

nationality, class and religion, and new identities emerging from fluid social networks.

Networked technologies offer several theoretical benefits to carers of people with dementia. In Castells' network society, we can see that tools such as the Internet can support the emergence of a carer identity. As a social group, carers, who have generally been relatively isolated individuals, often restricted in their movements by the needs of the person for whom they provide care, now have the means collectively to organise socially and politically. They have the potential to empower through enabling carers to become informed experts, providing access to knowledge and resources. Empowerment can also occur through peer-to-peer interactions, facilitating the sharing of information between carers. Networked technologies can provide psychosocial support, both in a formal, clinical sense with care services provided online and also through virtual communities of carers supporting each other. Such peer-to-peer interaction on the Internet can provide the support benefits identified in the (offline) large group work of Yalom and others – such as universality (knowing you are not alone), hope (knowing that there may be hope in a bad situation), the understanding and empathy of peers and the opportunity to be altruistic and to benefit from the altruism of others (Yalom 1995). A content analysis of messages posted to a US Alzheimer's disease email list in 2000 showed that this was used by family carers for information, sharing experiences and opinions and providing encouragement (White & Dorman 2000).

Other potential benefits of networked technologies include facilitating access to services – health, social and commercial. Carers of people with dementia are often socially isolated because of their geographical isolation, restricted by the need to constantly supervise the person with dementia. The Internet and related technologies can provide home access to health and social services, including remote consultations for both the carer and the person being cared for. It is known that both parties have unmet health needs which are partly due to the barriers they face in accessing formal health services.

One of the key features of networked technologies is that they allow instant transfer of data between geographical locations. Remote monitoring, whether by formal agencies or family carers, is another evolution from simple press button alarm systems to complex multisensor devices. This can include camera and sound monitoring allowing caring at a distance, perhaps monitored via the Internet or even on a mobile phone platform. It can also include developments in home health monitoring such as devices that check physiological function such as heart rate and blood pressure. If behaviour and/or health is surveyed remotely, this can ease restrictions on carer mobility. One particular issue in dementia care is that people with dementia can be prone to wandering, occasionally with tragic consequences. There are now devices that use satellite mapping technology to allow carers to identify the location of the individual they are caring for.

What were once considered simple 'stand-alone' assistive devices are increasingly being networked. The concept of the 'smart home' has been around for several years now, and expert systems are now allowing multiple devices in a household to become more joined-up, more intelligent and more available to consumers. So instead of merely assessing whether a tap has been left running, gas left on or an outside door left ajar, intelligent systems can now identify whether normal patterns of behaviour are being followed (e.g. by using pressure sensors or movement sensors to detect movement between rooms, from beds, from chairs, etc.) and to send alerts to carers if behaviour is sufficiently abnormal to fall outside the preset constraints of the system.

At the same time, the use of networked ICTs to support the caring role presents several potential threats. The first of these is digital exclusion – the fact that many carers who could benefit from a particular intervention will be excluded from doing so because they are unable to engage in the wired world of e-health. Carers of people with dementia often suffer financial hardship, and exclusion may be related to a lack of financial resources or may be because they lack, or perceive that they lack, the skills to use the new tools. We know that educational level corresponds strongly with Internet use (Dutton & Helsper 2007). It is also likely that those in higher socioeconomic groups are more able to access help with their computer use. Even if they do have access, and the ability to use the technology, accessibility issues related to poor eyesight or arthritic fingers may inhibit full engagement. Carers may also lack the level of 'e-health literacy' (Norman & Skinner 2006) required to make use of Web 2.0 initiatives such as social networking sites, which could help provide social support and reduce social isolation. That is, having not grown up immersed in such activity, they may lack the tacit knowledge to really exploit the potential of such initiatives.

Another threat of networked ICTs involves the real or perceived problems with digital abuse and misuse. In an interview study with mental health service users, we found that, although the biomedical world is obsessed with the quality of online health information, consumers themselves were much more concerned with misuse of virtual communities (Powell & Clarke 2007). Online interaction is perceived to be open to the risks of unregulated abusive and foul language and pornography, whether through deliberately targeted or random attacks.

Networked technologies can also lead to depersonalisation and dissociation. Depersonalisation describes the lack of human contact and the substitution of automation for interpersonal communication. Dissociation describes the loss of the local context. The nature of networks means they can facilitate communication across wide geographical areas, or even globally. They can allow people caring in the most unusual circumstances to find help or support from others in similar situations. Many people also value the anonymity that comes from such a distributed network. However, it can also mean that there is a loss of local context, and there is a question over whether individual social ties that are only established online can have the same strength as offline, local social ties.

Finally, networked technologies present several threats to privacy and autonomy. The scenarios of remote monitoring and intelligent systems described above may facilitate caring at a distance, allowing greater flexibility for carers who are often very constrained in their movements. At the same time, however, such benevolent surveillance can be seen as a threat to the privacy and autonomy of the person being cared for. Similarly, the autonomy of the carer can be threatened by an expert computer system that could take over their role. Caring for someone with dementia is known to be a very intense, very demanding experience. Sometimes, the metaphor of caring for a baby is used to describe how dependent the person with dementia is. However, although babies are highly dependent and demanding, and their lack of bladder and bowel control and irregular sleep patterns are shared with advanced states of dementia, when one is caring for infants, there is always the knowledge that the situation will improve, whereas in dementia care, the only real prospect is of gradual deterioration only ended by death. There seem to be two important coping mechanisms in such a situation. First, to have a predominant self-identity as a carer, and other roles are seen as secondary. Second, carers and the person they are caring for often see each other as sharing the problem of dementia: one of them has the symptoms, but they both have to cope with the problem together. As such, it is easy to see how systems that disrupt the caring role, with good intentions, can be seen as threats, and how carers can feel that it is also their privacy and autonomy that are eroded by external monitoring of the person with dementia.

While one can make arguments for both the potential benefits and the potential threats of new technology, and almost inevitably the truth will lie somewhere in between, there is also an argument that networked technologies may be both helpful and harmful at the same time. Burrows *et al.* (2000) highlighted the irony of rapid technological change creating both stress and isolation and at the same time being touted as the means of overcoming these problems. Based on an interview study with ten professional carers, Sävenstedt *et al.* (2006) described the 'duality in using information and communication technology in elder care', describing it as being a 'promoter of both inhumane and humane care'. Sävenstedt *et al.* (2006) described five dichotomies to illustrate this argument:

- Superficiality and genuineness
- Captivity and freedom
- Unworthiness and dignity
- Dissociation and involvement
- Threats and aids.

While relationships facilitated via ICTs can reduce the widespread isolation and loneliness of carers, they can also be seen to create a rather superficial reproduction of the closeness and intimacy of interpersonal relationships. Similarly, attempts to promote independent living, thus reducing the burden on carers, can at the same time promote captivity of the person being cared for – subject to various levels of intrusion through surveillance. This is linked to the concepts of 'unworthiness and dignity'. One aim of assistance through technology and the promotion of independence is the preservation of dignity, while also threatening that dignity through remote control and surveillance. From the carers' perspective, technology could support and extend their involvement, but could also lead to a certain physical and emotional disconnection in the relationship between carer and the person being cared for. Finally, Sävenstedt *et al.* (2006) describe carers being aware that, while new technologies may be helpful, they also present a threat to their role – that the introduction of such innovations could be seen as driven primarily by a desire to reduce costs rather than by health or social needs.

Intervention studies attempting to harness networked technology to support dementia carers

We know that traditional (non-computer) psychosocial support interventions for carers of people with dementia have the potential for some carers to improve psychological well-being (one systematic review identified this benefit in 15/25 studies which measured this, 60 per cent), improve caregiver burden (9/19 interventions, 47 per cent) and show improvements on measures of social support (5/14 interventions, 36 per cent) (Cooke *et al.* 2001). It is interesting that these results are far from conclusive and, clearly, interventions with components aimed at improving the quality or quantity of social contact have a variable effect on carers. Similarly, the evidence from intervention studies of online peer support (in general, not just for carers) is inconclusive when it comes to measuring the benefits of online peer support. A systematic review of this area (Eysenbach *et al.* 2004) found conflicting results for measures of depression, social support and health service utilisation, with the majority of studies finding no significant effects.

Given the potential benefits of new networked technologies in providing information and support to carers of people with dementia discussed above, it is interesting to review the studies that have attempted to evaluate such interventions. This section therefore takes an in-depth look at studies that specifically evaluated the value of networked ICTs for carers of people with dementia using some kind of comparative design. A short systematic review of the main findings from these studies has been published elsewhere (Powell *et al.* 2008).

There have been six studies of networked ICT interventions providing support to carers of people with dementia. This does not include studies that only looked at telephone support. We excluded these telephone studies as they did not provide services akin to Internet-based social interaction, whereas all the included studies did. The definition of networked technologies we used is probably closest to the older health informatics term of 'telematics', being the use of networked ICTs which permit the transfer of digital information between dispersed locations.

All the included studies were undertaken in North America. The first of these studies is the ComputerLink project run by Patricia Flatley Brennan and colleagues in Cleveland, Ohio (Brennan *et al.* 1995; Casper *et al.* 1995; Payton *et al.* 1995; Bass *et al.* 1998; McClendon *et al.* 1998). Brennan and colleagues gave carers the hardware and training to enable them to access a community computer network in the Cleveland area. ComputerLink provided carers with three functions: factual information via an electronic encyclopaedia aimed at promoting self-care; an online decision support module which used guided questioning to assist in the analysis of a self-defined problem; and communication via email, a public bulletin board (with nurse moderator) and a question and answer forum.

Although an early study using a community network rather than the global Internet, ComputerLink provided several of the functions now associated with Internet-based social interaction. The investigators undertook a randomised, controlled trial of 102 carers to assess its effectiveness on a range of outcome measures. Overall, the results showed that ComputerLink had little effect. While participants did demonstrate significantly improved confidence in decision-making, there was no overall improvement in decision-making skills, nor in measures of social support, perceived social isolation, carer strain, depression or health status. A common feature of these studies of networked interventions is that participants varied greatly in the intensity of use, and that average usage tended to be quite low. In ComputerLink, the average usage was twice per week, for 13 minutes per use. Carers used the interventions at all times of the day and night. The most frequently used functions were the communication ones, in particular posting messages on the forum. Carers reported that they valued the benefits of communication, companionship, interacting with others facing similar issues and being able to contact professionals for specific problems. They disliked having access problems when the system was being heavily used and having to remember email addresses. The messages posted by carers on the forum were most commonly related to mutual social support, information about the person with dementia's condition and the emotional impact of caring.

Three studies have been published from the large-scale Resources for Enhancing Caregiver Health (REACH) project (Mahoney *et al.* 2001; Czaja & Rubert 2002; Eisdorfer *et al.* 2003; Mahoney *et al.* 2003; Bank *et al.* 2006; Finkel *et al.* 2007). This project involved a collaboration of six separate research sites in the USA, investigating fifteen different interventions. The published studies describe two trials in Miami and one in New England. The REACH investigators in Miami tested a computer–telephone integrated system (CTIS) that provided menu-driven screen phones which used text and voice communication to access information on local services, conference calls to discussion groups, and send and receive voice and text messages (Czaja & Rubert 2002; Eisdorfer *et al.* 2003; Bank *et al.* 2006; Finkel *et al.* 2007). It was not a simple telephone intervention. In the first study of CTIS, they compared three groups each with about seventy-five participants: a minimal support control group, a group receiving family therapy and a group receiving both family therapy and the CTIS intervention (Czaja & Rubert 2002; Eisdorfer *et al.* 2003; Bank *et al.* 2006). They found that the last group receiving both CTIS and family therapy had improvements in depression scores, while the depression scores of the group receiving family therapy alone actually worsened. Carer satisfaction with CTIS was high. Eighty-one per cent of participants found the CTIS-based support groups to be of value in obtaining social and emotional support from other carers. The majority of carers also reported an increase in their knowledge and skills. Subsequently, Finkel and colleagues (2007) undertook a second, smaller randomised trial of CTIS, comparing this intervention alone with a minimal support group. In this small study with just twenty-three participants in each group, they found no differences in measures of social support, carer burden, depression or health behaviour (Finkel *et al.* 2007). There was an indication of improvements in depression scores for those who started the study more depressed but, as with all the studies described here, these *post hoc* analyses, often of small subgroups within the trials, need to be treated very cautiously.

The third published REACH study was undertaken by a different team working in New England (Mahoney *et al.* 2001, 2003). They also investigated a computerised telephone support system but with slightly differing features. This study was called REACH for Telephone Linked Care (TLC), and the menu-driven system provided a voicemail virtual support group designed to mimic a computer chat group, an automated stress monitoring and counselling interaction, voicemail messages to experts and peers and an automated respite call designed to be initiated by carers who would then use it to occupy and engage the person they were caring for. Again, this was not a simple telephone intervention, and it was designed with features mimicking Internet-based interaction. The authors carried out a randomised controlled trial comparing forty-nine participants given the system with a control group of fifty-one who only received an information booklet. The results showed no effect of the intervention in reducing measures of depression, anxiety or carer 'bother'. *Post hoc* subgroup analysis found that patients with lower mastery scores at baseline did show improvements on all three measures. Usage of the system was poor. Over the 12 months of the study, on average, each carer used the system for a total of 55 minutes. The investigators blamed this in part on poor system performance with several sporadic system failures. Non-adopters of the system also reported lack of relevance to their own situation as a reason for non-use.

Two more recent studies have evaluated Internet-based interventions. The first of these is AlzOnline, a study undertaken in Florida to evaluate the benefits of a package of Internet-based tools including psychoeducational classes, online library, frequently asked questions, links pages and a public message-board (Glueckauf & Loomis 2003; Glueckauf *et al.* 2004). In a very small pre- and post-test study with just twenty-one participants using the site for about 4 months, the investigators found some increases over the course of the intervention in measures of self-efficacy and perceptions of emotional burden. They found no differences in positive measures of the caring experience or in perceptions of time burden. The six psychoeducational classes were the main component of this intervention and could be accessed either via the Internet or by telephone if preferred. The investigators only report the findings from the twenty-one participants who completed the course of classes and do not provide an intention to treat analysis. Any estimate of effect is therefore likely to be an overestimate. In any case, the findings from such a small, uncontrolled study need to be treated with caution.

The final study was undertaken in Toronto, Canada. Marziali and colleagues (2006) tested the Caring for Others intervention, which provided Internet-based health information, a discussion forum, private messaging and both one-to-one and group video conferencing via a password-protected website. They carried out a randomised controlled trial over 6 months with three groups of carers: carers of people with Alzheimer's disease, with Parkinson's disease and with stroke (Marziali & Donahue 2006; Marziali *et al.* 2006). Thirty-four carers received the intervention, and thirty-two were in the no-intervention control group. Marziali and colleagues found that the website made no difference to carers on measures of social support, carer burden, depression or health status. They found a non-significant decline in stress in the intervention group compared with an increase in the control group. For an Internet-based intervention, this site was well used by carers with an average of 2.1 logins per day. The most popular feature was the disease-specific information, followed by private messaging and video conferencing. Over 90 per cent of carers found the virtual support group to be a positive experience, and 61 per cent felt that support obtained via online video conferencing was as helpful as face-to-face contact. Half the carers in the study had no prior experience of computer use, but 82 per cent of these reported feeling at least moderately comfortable with computer use after the study. The qualitative component of this study found that participants in the intervention valued the emotional benefits of online social interaction, particularly the empathy and understanding of other group members; the insights they gained into the management of their own thoughts and feelings; and help with the emotional reactions to the changing caring relationship including the possible transfer to institutional care. Again, the results of this study should be treated cautiously as it involves small numbers of participants and the drop-out rates were high (ten of the thirty-four members of the intervention group, and eighteen of the thirty-two in the control group did not complete the study).

Discussion

Carers of people with dementia bear a significant economic, social, psychological and physical burden. Their unpaid work subsidises the welfare state. Researchers at the University of Leeds working for the charity Carers UK estimate that the value of unpaid support provided by carers (not specifically caring for people with dementia) has now reached £87 billion a year (Carers UK 2007). This figure is similar to the annual NHS budget and four times the amount spent on adult and child social care services (Carers UK 2007). It is clear that new networked ICTs present theoretical benefits and harms for these carers. It is also clear that, with demographic change in an ageing population, the prevalence of chronic conditions such as dementia will increase, while the number of informal carers will diminish, as will the number of economically active adults contributing tax and national insurance. Telecare and related developments have been widely touted as possible solutions to the challenge presented by these social changes. Networked technologies in particular have been seen as having the potential to relieve social isolation and provide psychosocial support, as well as offering solutions such as teleconsultations, remote surveillance and intelligent monitoring systems.

With such innovation, there is always a danger of technological determinism, that the innovation drives and shapes social change. The needs of carers should come first, and technological solutions should support these needs. Not all carers will want to embrace networked technologies. Similarly, there are circumstances in which the prolonging of home-based care is not always a better option to institutionalisation. In this chapter, I have considered the theoretical threats and benefits from networked technology tools for carers. For the most part, these tools are being used to provide 'new ways of doing old things', for example providing social support, giving information and simply keeping an eye on the person being cared for. Two of the aspects of the new tools are their spatial and temporal flexibility – social support can come via synchronous or asynchronous communication in virtual communities with a global reach; expert information is available 24 hours a day at the anonymity of a home computer in the privacy of one's own house; audio and video surveillance can be undertaken from any location with network access. There are also ways in which the technology is facilitating new interactions, for example using intelligent systems in smart homes to monitor behaviour, potentially removing the carer role altogether until intervention is required.

The duality of new technology has been discussed, with reference to the impact of networked technologies on issues such as the nature of the caring relationship, the value of human contact, the importance of local context, the dignity and autonomy of the person being cared for. A recent paper by Robinson *et al.* (2007) described the need to balance 'risks and rights' in the surveillance of wandering in dementia care, where carers identified a conflict between the need, on the one hand, to minimise the risk of harm and, on the other, to minimise the threats to autonomy. Duality is also an important concept when discussing digital exclusion and the inequalities produced by new technology. Even if it does produce empowered, informed expert carers, it will also leave a group who are less empowered and less informed than some of their peers. There is also a danger in assuming that all carers want to embrace this information revolution, when some may wish to exclude themselves. In the digital divide of the have nets and the have nots, some of the have nots are quite content to be that way.

There have been a few attempts to evaluate the effectiveness of new networked ICT interventions in comparative studies. These have all been undertaken in North America, and all have involved complex interventions with various electronic features including encyclopaedic information, one-to-one communication, group discussion and sometimes with an element of decision support or psychoeducation. It is therefore difficult to determine the relative benefits of individual components such as peer support. Three of the six studies have come through the REACH project, which used a computerised text and voice telephone platform. This has usability advantages for a generation less accustomed to the home desktop computer user interface. One early study used a community computer network, a forerunner to the worldwide web. Two more recent studies evaluated Internet sites. In general, these evaluations have been carried out on relatively few participants, and usage rates of the interventions have often been poor. Drop-out rates in some of the studies have been high, and analyses were not all undertaken on an intention to treat basis. In addition, the majority of positive findings reported in the papers describing these studies have been based on subgroup analyses and should be treated cautiously. The generally poor quality of research in this area is also found in studies of telecare (Barlow *et al.* 2007). For the most part, the principal findings from these studies are inconclusive and certainly, taken as a whole, these research projects do not provide any consistent evidence for the beneficial effects of networked technologies in reducing social isolation or improving social support. However, they do not show harmful effects on either of these measures, and the subgroup analyses do at least suggest that certain carers had benefit.

Clearly, larger research studies would be useful to definitively test the hypotheses concerning the benefits of this technology. Inconclusive findings could be due to explanations other than the interventions being ineffective or the study size being too small to detect a real difference. The questionnaires used to measure characteristics such as social support may not be sensitive or specific enough for the outcome of interest, and constructs such as this are difficult to quantify. Outcomes such as empowerment were not consistently assessed and again are difficult to operationalise in a quantitative study. The qualitative components of these studies demonstrated that networked technologies are broadly acceptable to carers who generally reported high levels of satisfaction with them. However, this must of course be seen against the background of low usage.

A recent literature review of ICT as a support for frail older people living at home and their carers (not specifically related to caring for dementia) concluded that there is currently 'a dearth of studies that involve working together with frail older people and their family carers to search for new ICT solutions to meet their support needs' (Magnusson *et al.* 2004). As the early innovators in this area, the researchers undertaking the six studies reviewed in this chapter have been pioneering and, to some extent, have been driven by the possibilities of the technology at the time the research was undertaken, rather than by user needs and user ability. As such, the participants in these research studies have been required to be 'early adopters' of new technology, although that might not have come naturally to them. As the population becomes more accustomed to networked tools, and as these become available through a variety of platforms and more pervasive in the general environment, and particularly as the MySpace generation ages, the pool of carers with the tacit knowledge (the 'e-health literacy') to gain most benefit from such interventions will increase. However, there will still be pitfalls and barriers, and telecare should not be seen as a panacea for an ageing society in the twenty-first century. It will be important to keep the evaluation of the benefits of networked technologies for carers of people with dementia under review.

Notes

1 The review of intervention studies of networked information and communications technologies for carers of people with dementia is based on work undertaken for a systematic review with collaborators in Canada (Teresa Chiu and Gunther Eysenbach). This work was partly funded by a grant from the UK Department of Health Policy Research Programme.

Part III
Integrated user design

7 Making sense of sensors[1]

Older people's and professional caregivers' attitudes towards telecare

Julienne Hanson, Dorota Osipovič and John Percival

Introduction

This chapter explores the advantages and limitations of lifestyle monitoring (LSM) devices deployed in a telecare installation in an extra care housing setting for older people with impaired vision in south-west England, and discusses the attitudes and perceptions of the older people and their professional caregivers towards the technological devices that shared their homes and monitored their everyday lives. The uneasy relationship between people and technology is particularly exposed when it comes to issues relating to gerontechnology, that is, technology that is meant to support people in later life. Older people's attitudes towards such 'caring technologies' have hitherto not been sufficiently mapped. This account, which is based on the results of an 11-month-long telecare trial, synthesises feedback gathered from four rounds of in-depth interviews with six older participants, gauging their understanding of the technology and tracing their changing attitudes towards the sensors installed in their homes. These are compared with the findings from three rounds of interviews with seven professional care staff from the housing scheme, designed to detect the impact of telecare on their working lives and caregiving practices. Older people's attitudes towards various domestic objects bear heavily on their dispositions towards installed telecare devices, giving rise to a hierarchy of sensors that explains the varied degree of sensitivity and intrusiveness associated with sensoring different objects within the home environment. Moreover, as the case of the fall detector suggests, an immature and imperfect technology can even reverse the direction of the caring relationship, forcing older people to look after their troublesome devices. Although LSM proved capable of identifying changes in daily routines around the time of important health-related events, the retrospective interpretation of these changes required a large amount of contextual information and the involvement of the participants themselves. Furthermore, the findings to date highlighted technical and operational difficulties that need to be resolved before it will be possible to use LSM predictively.

Lifestyle monitoring

Telecare has been defined as the use of information and communications technology (ICT) to provide health and social care directly to the end-user, who may be either a patient or someone in need of care and support (Barlow *et al.* 2007). Interest in delivering ICT-based support and care to people living in their own homes has been stimulated in recent years by a rise in demand for such services resulting from the ageing society, coupled with government pressure to use resources more effectively by delivering more and better services with less money. The telecommunications sector has responded to these challenges by developing better underpinning technologies such as sensor design, information processing and user interfaces, while at the same time the more widespread uptake of ICT has led to a fall in the costs of telecommunications, thus making the service more attractive to providers.

Governments and health care providers in many parts of the world are therefore turning to telecare as a way of enhancing their existing support and care services. Within the UK, calls for telecare have been made in numerous government and other official documents since the late 1990s. At present, the UK has the highest demographic ratio of residents over the age of 65 in Europe (18.7 per cent), and the government plans to provide domestic assistive technology in the form of telecare by 2010 to people with disabilities or degenerative diseases who require this type of home-based care. More recently, the Department of Health has made over £100 million available (2006–9) to support new telecare service developments. Telecare is embedded in health policies relating to the management of chronic long-term ill-health and in moves to give patients greater choice over their care pathways, as well as in targets for reducing inappropriate admissions to and facilitating earlier discharges from hospital. It would seem to be here to stay.

One use of telecare is to monitor an individual's vital signs (heart rate, blood pressure, blood sugar level and the like), their safety and security in the home environment (through devices such as a smoke detector, flood detector or carbon monoxide detector) or their activities of daily living (such as moving about the home or using domestic equipment) through the use of sensor technology. This allows a response to be made in real time to a sudden change for the worse in an individual's vital signs, or if an emergency such as a flood or a fall is detected by the devices that monitor safety and activity in the domestic environment. In these situations, telecare is operating in an active mode, building on existing models of emergency or community alarm services. Many trials of home telecare have been undertaken to demonstrate its efficacy. One recent systematic review of telecare (Barlow *et al.* 2007) identified 8,666 papers reporting on the outcomes of telecare projects in scientific journals. Most of these focused on either vital signs monitoring or safety and security monitoring.

However, an alternative approach is to gather and analyse information over a long period of time from an array of sensors located throughout the home environment, in order to detect changes and trends in an individual's pattern of everyday activity. This form of passive monitoring, known as LSM, has attracted a great deal of interest because changes in lifestyle could signal deteriorating health, resulting in an increased need for care. LSM sensors monitor people's domestic routines and daily activities such as movement around the house, bed and chair occupancy, opening cupboards, doors, fridges and wardrobes, and use of various electrical devices such as kettles, TVs and lamps. Users are not required to wear any of the devices as they are positioned on the various objects in the home, so it is unobtrusive and avoids the problem that some people may reject wearable devices.

The idea behind LSM is that, by constant passive monitoring of the domestic environment through these various devices and by integrating them into an 'intelligent' LSM system, it will be possible to learn people's normal habits and routines and then to recognise, spot and keep track of significant deviations from this norm. Some deviations may be interpreted as signs of a forthcoming crisis, in which case, upon detecting them, an alert can be issued to a caregiver. Therefore, the ultimate aim of LSM is to provide more timely intervention in the event of an emerging crisis, by spotting small, accumulating signals suggestive of deteriorating well-being. This preventative approach is in line with the government's emphasis on self-care and lifelong health and well-being. One aim of the trial reported here was to evaluate the viability of LSM devices and to assess the potential for such predictive usage.

Some LSM trials have already been undertaken, and many claims have been made for its successful use, but data are unreliable. The research on which this chapter is based therefore brought together three universities, an NHS Foundation Trust, a specialist housing and care provider and a telecare supplier to investigate the challenges of introducing LSM in different types of housing setting and with different user groups. A key aim of the larger project, which took place between October 2003 and March 2007, was to test the potential of health and LSM to improve the independence of older people and their caregivers living in a range of housing environments (Barlow *et al*. 2005; Brownsell *et al*. 2006a, b; Percival & Hanson 2006; Hanson *et al*. 2007b; Laviolette & Hanson 2007). This chapter focuses on the findings from one such environment, an extra care housing scheme for older people with impaired vision located in the south-west of England.

Living independently in a home of one's own is an objective that most older people wish for, but achieving this takes on added significance for people who are visually impaired, as moving from a well-known location to an unfamiliar one can be disorienting and distressing. This is especially so when impaired vision is compounded by chronic health conditions such as high blood pressure, diabetes or epilepsy. A trial telecare service was therefore established in the homes of six older people with such conditions in order to explore the potential benefits in promoting independent living, managing long-term conditions more proactively and improving quality of life.

Lifestyle monitoring in an extra care setting

The 11-month trial took place between January and November 2006. After several consultation meetings held during the autumn of 2005, six older participants were recruited to the trial (Table 7.1). The group comprised four women and two men; four people were in their 80s, one in his 40s and one in her 60s. Five lived alone and one lived with her husband and a guide dog. Five out of the six participants had vision impairment and one person had both severe vision and hearing impairment. All six had other serious health conditions.

The flats in the extra care scheme occupied by the research participants were all different, so a detailed floor plan of each flat was prepared, taking account of the positioning of the furniture, in order to accurately position the sensors installed in each participant's flat so that all relevant daily activity would be recorded. The sensors in each flat were carefully chosen to reflect aspects of each participant's lifestyle, routine and habits. In Miss Evans' flat, which had a typical array of sensors, sixteen sensors were installed altogether comprising five passive infrared movement detectors (PIRs; marked as black triangles), a bed occupancy sensor, a bed epilepsy sensor, a chair occupancy sensor, three electric usage sensors on the TV, kettle and little oven and five door contact sensors on the wardrobe, fridge-freezer, kitchen cupboard, bathroom cupboard and front door (Figure 7.1).

An average of 14.8 different sensors was installed in each of the six flats (Table 7.2). In contrast with telecare devices operating in an active mode that raise a real time alert in response to an emergency situation, the LSM devices listed in Table 7.2 operated in a passive mode by continuously monitoring each participant's activity within the home. The data gathered by the

Table 7.1 Participants' characteristics

Pseudonym of participant	Gender	Age (years)	Household composition	Health conditions
Mrs Adams	Female	80	One person household	Vision impairment, hypertension, diabetes
Mrs Bishop	Female	68	Married couple household	Vision impairment, hypertension
Miss Evans	Female	84	One person household	Vision impairment, hearing impairment, coronary heart disease, epilepsy
Mr Gibson	Male	82	One person household	Vision impairment, hypertension, diabetes, cancer
Mr Heaton	Male	47	One person household	Vision impairment, cerebral palsy, hypertension
Mrs Jenkins	Female	84	One person household	Diabetes, coronary heart disease

Table 7.2 Summary of sensors installed in the flats

Sensors	Mrs Adams	Mrs Bishop	Miss Evans	Mr Gibson	Mr Heaton	Mrs Jenkins	Total
Bed occupancy	1	0	1	1	0	1	4
Chair occupancy	2	0	1	0	0	1	4
Door usage	4	4	4	4	7	4	27
Electrical usage	3	4	3	4	4	4	22
Movement (PIRs)	5	6	5	5	5	6	32
Total	15	14	14	14	16	16	89

Note: PIR, passive infrared movement detectors.

individual devices and sensors were transmitted via a home hub, through a server installed on site and eventually to the researcher's computer at the university. All analysis of this data stream was done retrospectively and not in real time. Meanwhile, the participants continued to use the community alarm in the extra care setting to summon assistance in the event of a real emergency.

In addition to the LSM, all six participants were given fall detectors, which had to be worn round the waist, and two participants at their own request received talking blood pressure monitors. These two individuals measured their blood pressure themselves, whereas for the other four participants, blood pressure measurement was performed regularly once or twice a week by the housing scheme's staff, according to a protocol that had been agreed in advance with the help of the local community nurse. Three participants also had their blood sugar regularly monitored in this way. This and other information was regularly logged onto health monitoring sheets, which also served as diaries for logging the dates of any relevant events, such as holidays or hospitalisations, in the lives of the participants.

The research team used a mixed research methodology that included in-depth interviews, health monitoring and events diaries, as well as mining the data streams emerging from the sensors installed in participants' homes. Four rounds of in-depth interviews were conducted with the older participants. The main aim of the initial, pre-installation interview was to collect contextual information about participants' daily routines and activities, in order to specify an appropriate package of LSM. The second round took place about 6 weeks after telecare had been installed and recorded participants' early experiences of the service. A third round of interviews was conducted after 9 months to record longer term experiences of living with LSM, and a final round of interviews took place shortly after the removal of the sensors to record participants' considered reflections on the whole experience.

Seven members of staff from the extra care setting, representing all levels from care assistants to senior support workers and the scheme manager, were interviewed in November 2005 before the packages of LSM were installed, in March 2006 to gauge the early impact of the installation on staff morale and working practices, and in December 2006, after the devices had been removed

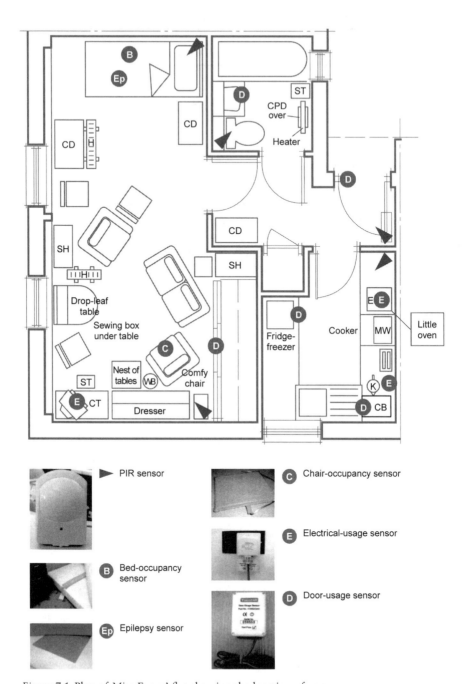

Figure 7.1 Plan of Miss Evans' flat showing the location of sensors

from participants' flats. Each interview consisted of two parts: a semi-structured interview based on a topic guide followed by a 'perceived stress scale' that asked staff to assess the impact of the project on key aspects of their workload (upset, loss of control, nervousness and stress, confidence, advantages and benefits, inability to cope, irritation, feeling on top of the job, anger and diffi-culties piling up) on a scale from one to five, where one represented that they were 'never' affected and five that they were 'very often' affected in this way by the telecare trial. The topics addressed by staff included their thoughts about its impact on working practices at the extra care scheme, the good and not so good aspects of LSM, the impact it had on their interaction with the tenants and the contact staff had with local general practitioners (GPs) and other health care professionals as a result of the trial. The project received ethics approval from both UCL's Research Ethics Committee and the relevant Local NHS Research Ethics Committee.

Caregivers' perspectives on telecare

Care staff from the extra care setting reported that tenants had initially been very anxious about the trial, with concerns about the devices possibly affecting their privacy or undermining their sense of independence, but that these fears and anxieties gradually settled down in the first few weeks of the trial. In this respect, staff explained that visually impaired older people might have been particularly sensitive to technology that was unfamiliar because they could not familiarise themselves with it through sight, and it might therefore seem more worrying or more of an intrusion because of this.

Staff confirmed that the telecare project had made little impact on their day-to-day work, other than that this had led to checking the blood pressure of some tenants. This work was seen as an extra element of support that had been easily absorbed and soon constituted a routine activity among others. Blood pressure monitoring was seen as an effective way of unobtrusively gau-ging a tenant's state of well-being, especially important in respect of those people who were not inclined to say they were unwell or to ask for help. Indeed, several care and support staff emphasised that the monitoring of tenants' blood pressure should continue as a regular task, given its pre-ventative role in health care and the positive feedback staff had received from relevant tenants. One or two examples were provided of tenants whose medi-cation had been changed quickly as a result of blood pressure readings repor-ted by staff, and this had endorsed the value of this work for staff as well as the positive impact of their new 'telecare' role.

Staff unanimously agreed that the project had not affected their job com-plexity and in many ways their role had 'stayed the same', thus relieving any anxieties that telecare would reduce the need for face-to-face contact with caregivers. There had been little for staff to engage with as regards the LSM, partly because the data generated by the devices installed in tenants' flats were directed elsewhere and partly because the tenants had not engaged with the fall detectors, the only piece of equipment likely to demand staff attention. There was very little variation in the responses to the carers' perceived stress scale throughout the telecare trial, suggesting that staff continued to experience little or no stress as a result of the project. Indeed, most interviewees acknowledged that the project had not caused any significant change to their work and had little or no impact on their daily routines.

Some interviewees reflected that they had learned the importance of introducing telecare, particularly the technological aspects, in a sensitive way that minimised service users' concerns. In this respect, staff said that relevant professionals needed to be 'empathetic' to prospective service users because it appeared that telecare could make some people 'think about their disabilities' to the extent that it reduced self-esteem. Telecare providers therefore needed to understand how telecare might be perceived by service users in order to allay their fears and reiterate clear and accurate information.

Aspects of the project that were well received included collaboration with other professionals involved with the trial, the additional health monitoring of tenants through checking their blood pressure readings and the expectation that, given this health monitoring in the extra care setting, 'surgery time' had been saved, allowing district nurses and others to attend to more acute tasks. The word 'reassurance' was used a number of times by interviewees to describe the effect of the project in general and the deployment of additional health monitoring, through blood pressure checks, in particular. Staff felt reassured that they were providing closer, more proactive scrutiny of vulnerable tenants by having telecare modifications *in situ*.

However, there was a tendency for some interviewees to get carried away by the prospect of an all-seeing, benevolent LSM system, which could 'inform us' when someone left their fridge door open by mistake. Although this perception of telecare's role was rather unrealistic, it indicated the general enthusiasm of staff for a LSM service that could alert caregivers to cases of self-neglect or worrying behaviour. Notwithstanding these positive views, interviewees also raised their disappointment at certain shortcomings of the technology, especially the unreliability of certain devices and the possible loss of potentially valuable data due to equipment failure. Staff also regretted the lack of take-up of the fall detectors, and speculated that such devices have to be better designed and targeted to be accepted by older service users.

The interviews revealed that, for some, LSM may have been a mixed blessing in that, while it offered reassurance to tenants, it was also perceived as a process that accentuated their neediness and deficits and, in the case of some participants, it drew attention to their need for additional help in a more public way because of the ever present monitoring devices. This more negative perception could perhaps prevent some people from recognising the actual or potential benefits of telecare. Staff indicated that, for these reasons, the providers of telecare services should acknowledge that people's acceptance of help through such services may be problematic and should pay careful attention to individuals' sensitivity on this matter, especially in respect of safeguarding a sense of independence. Staff also raised the point that some tenants continued to be anxious about the surveillance potential of LSM, even after it had been repeatedly explained that the devices did not record any visual images of their activities.

Participants' attitudes and motivations

Unlike the care staff, who tended to share similar attitudes to telecare, the participants split into two groups on three important dimensions, with regard to their general attitudes towards technology, their preference for active or passive participation and their expectations about the research (Table 7.3). Like other studies (Fisk 2003), this LSM trial contradicted the popular view that older people are technophobes. On the contrary, three participants could be described as technophiles, while the attitude of the other three towards technology in their everyday life was indifferent but not hostile. One of the technophiles, Mr Gibson, pointed out that he had served in the RAF during the war, which explained his positive attitude towards technology. He added, 'They hadn't got the technical aids then that they've got now, I agree, but they were quite technical. I remember using radar for the first time'. Another technophile, Mr Heaton, described himself as 'a bit of a gadget person', while the only woman among the technophiles, Mrs Bishop, noted 'I like taking things to bits and putting them back together again. I've always had to do it all me life'. On the other hand, participants indifferent to technology listed many assistive technology devices for people with impaired vision, such as a talking clock, mug and the like, that they used on a regular basis. Their overall attitude towards technology was best described by one participant who said, 'I'm quite happy with what I've got and my way of living'.

These general attitudes towards technology had an impact on how involved in the research process our participants wanted to be. Again, the group split in half, into those who wanted to have a hands-on approach to the project and

Table 7.3 Participants' attitudes to technology

General attitudes to technology in everyday life	
Technophiles	*Indifferent*
Mrs Bishop, Mr Gibson, Mr Heaton	Mrs Adams, Miss Evans, Mrs Jenkins
Preference for participation	
Hands-on	*Hands-off*
Mrs Bishop, Mr Gibson, Mr Heaton	Mrs Adams, Miss Evans, Mrs Jenkins
Expectations of research benefits	
Self-oriented	*Others-oriented*
Mrs Bishop, Mr Heaton, Miss Evans	Mrs Jenkins, Mr Gibson, Mrs Adams

those who limited their role to being helpful but remaining in the background. The latter group explicitly requested that they should not be overwhelmed with information about the trial and all the intricacies and complexities of the research, whereas the enthusiasts expected feedback to be provided on a more or less continuous basis. Mr Heaton was particularly enthusiastic about the research, 'I think it's going to be interesting for me as well ... So this would be like a new thing to like see how it goes, you know I'm quite interested in it, to find out a bit more as we go along. ... I'm very interested how it's going to come, what the results is going to be'.

Finally, a clear difference was observed when it came to the participants' expectations about the results of the trial, which could be classified into either 'self-oriented', in that they expected to draw some direct benefits for their personal life situation, or 'others oriented', for those participants who embraced the spirit of the research because, although it would probably not benefit them directly, it might benefit other people in the future. Mrs Bishop and her husband, representing the self-oriented attitude, voiced their concern about the research not being useful to them personally in the following statement, 'At first the idea of having different equipment around seemed quite good but that was until we've seen it all. Half of the stuff would be no use to us and we've raised this issue at the beginning of the project'. On the other hand, Mrs Jenkins and Mr Gibson held a strongly opposed view, which helped them persevere throughout the research. As Mrs Jenkins observed, 'Sometimes it annoys me seeing all these ... like the thing under my cushion and under my bed, but these don't worry me because I think, well if it helps understand, perhaps in future generations it might be a help to somebody'. The importance of noting these attitudinal differences is that, when extended to the wider community, the same package of telecare may provoke different responses, depending on these more general attitudes to and expectations about the role of technology within society.

Living with lifestyle monitoring

In the early stages of the trial, participants were encouraged to express their understanding of the research and their role in it. The aim of this was to check the efficiency of the communication process undertaken in preparation for the project and to uncover any areas of misunderstandings. Generally, at the outset, participants were not entirely sure what 'participation' would entail. This uncertainty related to the type and function of the devices that they had been offered, as Mrs Bishop explained, 'Well to be honest with you I'm not too sure, I've got to be honest about this. I know we were talking about something for people that fall. We were talking about blood pressure monitoring. And I know you said you might have a problem with doing the infrared things in the house because of the dog'.

Crucially, some participants had a problem in understanding that the LSM devices would operate in a passive and not in an active response mode. This resulted in statements such as the ones below by Mrs Adams, 'It's there to keep an eye on me ... ', and elsewhere in the same interview, 'With the thing up in the corner it's watching me, so if I was to fall or anything like that then it would alarm'. These misplaced assumptions on the part of most participants about the passive response mode of LSM sensors such as the PIRs led them to experience an increased level of anxiety about causing unnecessary alerts and therefore burdening support staff. The message that LSM was operating in a passive mode had to be repeated on a number of occasions before participants' concerns about generating false alerts was put to rest.

A hierarchy of sensors

Longer term, participants' attitudes towards specific sensors could be summarised by looking at their perceived intrusiveness. It soon became apparent that certain domestic objects were infused with a greater degree of intimacy and privacy than others. What followed from this was that the participants objected strongly to the instrumenting of intimate objects, while at the same time they took an indifferent position when it came to instrumenting less emotionally charged objects. This reaction suggested that there was an underlying hierarchy of sensors (Figure 7.2) that was generated from unspoken rules that the older participants were applying to rank the different sensors according to their perceived or real intrusiveness. This proposition was tested and confirmed by asking each participant to rank each type of sensor on a scale from one (not at all intrusive) to five (very intrusive).

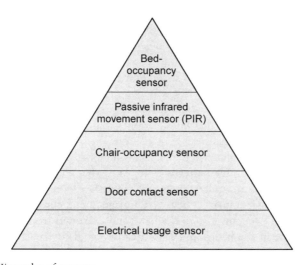

Figure 7.2 Hierarchy of sensors
Note: The base of the pyramid shows the least intrusive and its tip the most intrusive type of sensor.

The sensors that our participants found least problematic were electric usage sensors fitted on kettles, lamps, TVs and other electrical appliances. Door contact sensors have been placed on the next level up from the least intrusive sensors. The main concerns voiced by the participants with regard to door contact sensors were of a functional nature. Participants complained that the sensors were bulky, they upset the balance of fridge and cupboard doors and, as Mrs Bishop put it, they, 'kept falling off, it was getting in the way'. Half the participants reported problems with the chair occupancy sensor. This was either because the chair sensor could not be fitted to the participant's chair or because it made the chair uncomfortable to use. Complaints about the chair occupancy sensor were also related more to design and functionality than to its intrusion into the intimate aspects of people's domesticity. As Mr Gibson stated, 'It was giving me back ache, this is a recliner anyway and it was completely putting me off and I was sliding forward all the time'. Miss Evans explicitly differentiated her attitudes towards her chair sensor from the much more intrusive issue of her bed sensor, 'I can cope with my chair. ... I never felt the same as I felt about my bed'.

People's attitudes towards PIRs were more complex. One thing that bothered nearly all the participants was the issue of red lights, which flashed intermittently when movement was detected. The red light was unacceptable to many participants with various vision impairment conditions. Mrs Bishop expressed the predominant view, 'It kept coming on in the bathroom with the light, it kept coming on, and I could not stand that, I did not know what it was'. This aspect of PIR operation was subsequently suppressed. However, stopping the flashing lights led to another problem, namely the lack of any feedback mechanism within these devices that would enable the user to check whether they were actually working. People struggled to understand the passive principle behind the operation of the PIRs and failed to find an answer to what the PIRs were doing in their homes. Although the whole LSM installation was operating in a passive mode, the PIRs seemed to be singled out in a negative way by the participants as embodying this passive principle. Therefore, the functionality of the PIRs was not easily understood compared with that of other types of sensor deployed in the installation. It continued to be regarded with suspicion as surveillance rather than assistive technology, which was reminiscent of 'Big Brother'.

Before the flashing lights were switched off, some participants appeared to be searching for discernible patterns to explain what caused the PIRs to flash, possibly in search of an understanding of what they were actually monitoring about the home environment. They were intrigued and curious, as Mr Gibson explained, 'I don't see any reaction when I move around from that one, like I do with the one in the bedroom'. Miss Evans was also puzzled by the operation of the PIRs in her home, 'When I get out of my chair then I get nearly to the door and the light either comes off or goes on, it flashes or something. Because I'm busy coming this way I don't see them. I don't know which one of them it is. That might be my wardrobe of course'.

Beds proved to be the most emotionally charged items of furniture and so instrumenting the bed caused a considerable upheaval for three of the six participants. In two cases, the bed sensors were subsequently removed. The third person, despite voicing her concern, did not wish the sensor to be removed. Objections to the bed sensor could be boiled down to issues of privacy, dignity and sexuality. In addition, in the case of Miss Evans, the introduction of an epilepsy bed sensor significantly altered this participant's existing coping strategies.

The installation of the epilepsy sensor was a traumatic experience for Miss Evans, who went on from a stage of crisis, withdrawal and defiance to a state of rationalisation and acceptance of her new situation. Initially, her sleep pattern became significantly disrupted, 'I just couldn't go to bed that night and I went over ... I just want to run away, run out of my flat now, there's nowhere left. And that's how I felt'. Later, Miss Evans expressed views that revealed her growing acceptance of the fact that she will become less independent with the passage of time, 'I look at it as if they're trying to help me because I'm older, it's the only way I can and it doesn't matter. Although it was a mini hurdle to get over'. Miss Evans gradually redefined her whole situation so that it became easier for her to accept the sensor in her bed.

For many of our participants, as for Miss Evans, the bed was an object saturated with intimate meanings and feelings, 'My bed was where I could relax and be comfortable, curl up and think fine, you know, I'm here, that's it'. Her bed was a place of refuge which, in addition, for this particular person, was also a place were she felt 'in control' of her epilepsy. Seen in this light, it is easy to understand how invasive the installation of an epilepsy bed sensor must have been for this participant. This serves to remind us that the installation of a particular sensor may trigger an outburst of associations and memories and could even destroy a fragile pre-existing structure of various tested ways of coping with the condition that the sensor is meant to support. It may also require developing new ways of coping with the condition the sensor is meant to monitor. Unfortunately, advice on the best ways of doing so does not come together with the sensor operation manual.

Mr Heaton, the youngest participant, while voicing his objections, touched on the issue of sexuality. His bed was fitted with two bed occupancy sensors, one on each side of his double bed. Shortly afterwards, he asked for them to be removed. During the follow-up interview, he elaborated on his objections to the devices in his bed, 'Well just say if you had a girlfriend with you, right you could tell that you've got two of us in the bed because the pads were alarmed and I wouldn't want that. ... For a young person and I thought really why should I tell somebody on the end of a computer what time I get up, what time I go to bed. That I found distressing. The things in the room because you're up, that didn't bother me but when I went to bed I thought, they've got all the information but sometimes you still need a bit of privacy'. As beds are one of the most intimate objects in the home, if not the most intimate, one should be extremely careful when offering a package of LSM that includes a bed sensor.

On the other hand, it has to be said that, even in the case of this most intrusive sensor, three participants did not have any objections, so Mrs Adams remarked of her bed sensor, 'They're not interfering with me, so I mean they've been put there, so I mean as far as I'm concerned they can stay there, unless they want to come and uproot it and take it out'. Mrs Jenkins concurred, 'My bed, no I can't say I notice any difference'. So did Mr Gibson, 'I did feel it there, I know it's there but it doesn't inconvenience me at all, not like the one in the chair'. These highly individualised reactions towards various sensors suggest that, when trying to tailor a set of appropriate devices to an individual's needs, one should consider not only the more obvious social and health variables such as age or health conditions but also the more elusive variable of personality, as just how much intrusion a person is prepared to accept depends on their personality and many other factors. Furthermore, telecare providers need carefully to 'unpack' any so-called 'package of sensors' because devices that are generally perceived to be non-intrusive (such as a flood detector) or even helpful (such as a blood pressure monitor) may be packaged together with devices that, for some individuals, are highly charged with significant meanings or downright dysfunctional. In this sense, portraying a set of telecare devices with different degrees of functionality and acceptability as a uniform, value-free and operationally integrated package may even be misleading.

Taking care of technology

People experienced individual reactions to specific sensors but, over and above this, the main change in participants' attitudes towards technology during the research related to the process of getting used to the whole array of LSM devices installed in their homes. In particular, because of the passive mode of their operation, they became somewhat 'invisible'. Mrs Jenkins echoed the views of other participants about the 'invisibility' of the installed sensors, 'sometimes I forget they're there. I mean I know there's something under the cushion, I know there's something under my bed but I don't often think about it and it's only when you come that I really remember that it's there'. However, technology operating in the background is not always a good thing when it comes to the issue of checking whether the equipment is working and the lack of a feedback mechanism. As Mrs Bishop observed, 'it does not tell us nothing, we assume that it is working but we don't know. So there is no way for us to know whether the equipment is working and whether it does what it is meant to do'. Knowing whether equipment is working and having the possibility of testing it is crucial, particularly in those situations where the whole support system is built around a piece of technological equipment.

Generally, over the course of the monitoring period, which was only 11 months, many problems relating to mending and servicing the equipment emerged. This applied to all the installed devices. Participants reported the need to fix devices that fell off the walls or doors or tighten those fitted too loosely. The issue of changing the batteries in equipment was also mentioned on two occasions. One can argue that, in the second half of the project, participants spontaneously involved themselves in a process of 'looking after' the equipment, which is an inversion of the caring relationship as it was supposed to look after them. The unreliability of devices also adversely affected the care staff at the scheme, as reported earlier.

The double life of the fall detector

All six participants were given fall detectors to wear. However, it soon became clear that only one out of the six participants, Mr Heaton, was prepared to use it and even so he was not entirely happy with the design and functionality of the fall detector. The fall detector used in this trial had to be worn on a belt around the waist. It detected a fall by measuring both the strength of an impact and the angle at which the device came to rest. When a fall was detected, the fall detector emitted a signal, which, if not deactivated by the user within a certain time limit, was sent to a response centre. In this case, the alarm went to the support worker on duty in the extra care setting in which our participants were living. This was the only instance of a sensor (other than the epilepsy sensor, discussed earlier) that operated in active mode.

The fall detector used on this particular trial was quite sensitive. Our participants were therefore worried about causing unnecessary alerts and putting an extra burden on support staff. This fear might also be explained by the fact that, when falling is an issue, older people perceive the potential risk to their social identity as being greater than the physical risk of falling. On the other hand, health professionals are mainly concerned with managing physical risk associated with falling. Our participants were concerned that causing too many false alarms might endanger their status with regard to the support staff, putting them in an 'at risk' category, and that eventually this might even endanger their housing situation, with a threat of moving to residential care if they seemed to fall too often.

Mrs Adams recalled an episode when a false alarm was caused, 'And of course trying [to put it on] mine fell on the floor. Of course the office came running to see if I was all right and all that business you see. ... I didn't think that was fair because you see, we're over stretched with staff, the same as everywhere else'. Miss Evans was equally concerned about the issue of false alarms, 'It made me nervous over there because he said if you knock it over it would beep, well I only go to do my shoes up and the thing beeped ... and therefore I didn't know what to do with it. ... I come down to do my shoes and it's at that angle ... ... so I have to be sure that's somewhere else you know ... I mean I haven't had many emergencies, not really, I haven't beeped really'.

In addition to the issue of false alarms, participants complained about the bulkiness of the device itself, that it was uncomfortable to wear, that it could not be used at night when arguably it was most needed, and that it was difficult for a person with vision impairment to operate. Furthermore, there was also a gender issue in that women, who do not wear belts, found it particularly bulky and impractical. Mrs Adams voiced the concerns of the female participants, 'I don't have a belt or anything like that you see and seeing that I have to have my alarm there you see and the key's on top of the skirt, you see I mean it's a bit cumbersome. Like I say I don't really need it'. Mrs Bishop even worried about the potential harm that wearing a fall detector might cause her, 'When you wear it around the waist you can do yourself more harm if you fall on your side, on your hip, and the fall detector would squeeze up against your stomach. I haven't worn it. It's too cumbersome'.

It has become common knowledge that objects tend to acquire 'a life of their own'. Although it is human actors who infuse things with their socially constructed meanings and purposes, one can only see the changes in these meanings through focusing on the objects themselves rather than human agency, and by tracking objects' 'adventures' through times and places (Appadurai 1986). Objects can be infused with new meanings, and new uses for such objects can be invented; in extreme cases, the initial functionality of the object may be turned upside down. In this respect, the work of Mihaly Csikszentmihalyi and Eugene Rochberg-Halton who have researched the role of domestic objects in the identity formation processes (Csikszentmihalyi & Rochberg-Halton 1981) comes to mind. In their research, these authors advanced a distinction between action and contemplation objects and activities. Action activities embrace people's interactions with objects on a physical or kinetic level, whereas contemplation activities describe people's engagement with the objects primarily on a mental level. The results of their research into cherished domestic objects provide us with ample examples of objects that, in the course of people's lives, have made a transformation from being an object used primarily for action activities to objects that became the focus of contemplation activities.

In respect of the fall detectors, a strong desire to avoid false alarms and not to attract the attention of the staff, combined with the perception of the fall detector as 'a very sensitive thing', resulted in participants' going to great lengths in looking after their unloved and unused fall detectors. From a typical action object, the essence of which lies in kinetic principles of movement through the bending and falling that it is suppose to monitor, fall detectors were transformed into static, motionless ornaments, representatives of the family of objects called bric-a-brac. As with the PIRs, this reversed the original relationship that people were meant to establish with their fall detectors from a device that provided reassurance and looked after them to an object that one should look after, be careful with and keep an eye on because of its sensitive nature (Hanson & Osipovič 2007; Osipovič & Hanson 2007; Figure 7.3).

All the participants made sure that their fall detectors were placed in an upright position and in what they called a 'safe' place. Miss Evans put her fall detector on the display cabinet. Mrs Bishop also kept her fall detector on the display cabinet and stated, 'It is on the display cabinet so grandchildren can't reach it and knock it over'. Mrs Adams tucked hers away in the corner of the

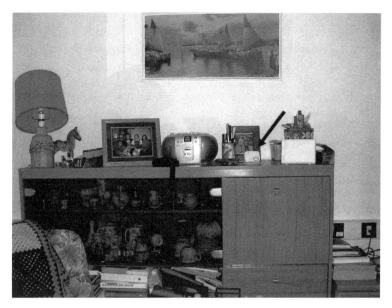

Figure 7.3 Location of Miss Evans' fall detector

windowsill, 'It's on the windowsill, why have it if it keeps falling on the floor and alarming everybody'. Mr Gibson kept his fall detector on the coffee table in the living room 'standing upright'. He noted somewhat ironically, 'This system here, as I say is lying quite comfortably out there, absolutely no use to me'. During the next visit, he added, 'I always make sure that it is normally safe'. Mrs Jenkins neither liked nor used her fall detector but could not recall where she put it in her home. The only person who liked the idea of a fall detector and was prepared to 'give it a go', Mr Heaton, kept his fall detector on his medicine table. This placement was also meaningful as, in contrast with the previously shown placement of useless fall detectors, in this case, the fall detector was perceived as having useful, almost medicinal and curing qualities. To summarise, efforts to keep the fall detector in an 'upright' and static position were related to concerns about setting it off accidentally. Such efforts signified the inversion of the relationship of care. Paradoxically, by 'fixing' the fall detectors on display cabinets and tables, our participants were ultimately trying to prevent the fall detectors from falling (Figure 7.4).

In contrast with opinions about the fall detector, the feedback on the blood pressure monitoring received by participants was generally very positive. Two participants who received their own talking blood pressure monitors were particularly fond of this device and described it as 'brilliant'. The talking blood pressure monitor ticked all the boxes with our participants in that it had all the essential features of user-centred design; it was interactive, responsive and easy to use, it left the control over the device entirely in the user's hands and enabled blood pressure to be measured independently without help from other people and without the need to go to the GP's surgery, 'The blood pressure monitoring was the most useful, it was God sent, my GP was impressed, I am doing it myself, regularly'. The talking feedback it provided was particularly important for people with impaired vision who could not read a visual display.

Whereas both participants equally appreciated their talking blood pressure monitors, they took opposite views when it came to sharing this device with other people or keeping it just for their own private use. Mrs Bishop was very protective of her device, 'I do it pretty regularly, normally I take it twice just to make sure and I am not "lending" it to anyone', whereas Mr Gibson remarked, 'it is a personal thing to me but on the other hand my neighbours will come in sometimes and check theirs, I'm the community nurse'. Mr Gibson's experience suggests that possessing such a useful piece of equipment can elevate someone's status in the neighbourhood, strengthen their social networks and facilitate sociability. However, had the trial been 'live' and in the community, sharing the blood pressure monitor around would almost certainly have confused any health care professional who tried to interpret the various readings.

Maybe it is not so surprising that the older people on the LSM trial assumed a caring role for the devices that were introduced into their homes, as ensuring order in the domestic environment is a way of taming and controlling the

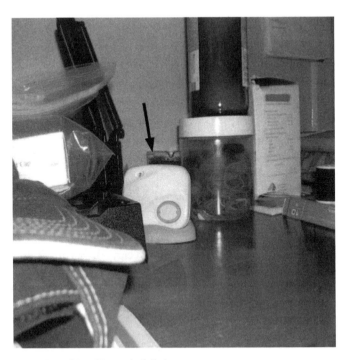

Figure 7.4 Location of Mr Heaton's fall detector

living space that humans inhabit and engage with on a daily basis. From a product design perspective, it should be made easier for people to look after their devices and for the devices to look after people. This research has shown the importance of placing control over the device in the hands of end-users. Moreover, the users of telecare may not necessarily view passive monitoring as a more satisfactory solution than a system with which they can become actively engaged, and this provides a counter argument to the popular belief that the advantage of an LSM system over basic response mode telecare is that the users do not need to engage with the devices in any way. Both the success of the talking blood pressure monitor and the fact that this telecare trial made all the participants more appreciative of their existing alarm system, based on pendants and pull cords that have to be operated manually by the user, point in that direction.

Detecting deteriorating patterns of health

At the start of the telecare trial, it had been hoped that it would be possible to detect changes in observed patterns of sensor firings over a period of time, which would expose changes in an individual's everyday regime that were indicative of declining health. The intention behind this objective was to facilitate an early intervention, perhaps altering medication or adjusting diet before the individual's ill-health had reached crisis point. It had also been suggested that, in theory, an individual could be discharged early from hospital and sent home with a package of telecare that could monitor behaviour at home, alerting care providers to any negative changes to routine such as failure to eat regularly or to take medication, which could indicate that the person concerned was not managing independently in the community. In this manner, theoretically speaking, it ought to be possible both to prevent unnecessary hospital admissions and to facilitate earlier hospital discharges.

What the LSM trial uncovered was that there are many difficulties in achieving this objective, which have to do with the way in which the data obtained from sensors are interpreted in order to detect any pattern in the flow of information. Even where the situation is a relatively straightforward one of a person living alone, allowing the information obtained from sensors to be directly attributed to an individual's actions, things that may interfere with the process of attribution include such factors as changes in medication that can alter the routine in ways that are not directly related to health.

The difficulties in assigning a preventative role to LSM can be illustrated by the case of Miss Evans, who was hospitalised for a 2-week period in March 2006 because of a sudden rise in her blood pressure. Retrospectively, the pattern of sensor firings in Miss Evans' home was intensively explored for the days leading up to her emergency hospitalisation and after she had been discharged (Hanson *et al.* 2007a). In the run-up to her hospitalisation, a slight increase in Miss Evans' blood pressure was recorded on her health monitoring sheets. Nevertheless, until the day of the crisis, all her blood pressure readings were within a range considered 'normal' for this individual, so health monitoring alone would not have led to an earlier, remedial intervention.

Retrospectively, a number of significant changes in the pattern of sensor firings were observed in the period leading towards hospitalisation, compared with the period after Miss Evans' return from hospital. Before hospitalisation, there was more bed sensor activity during the night time, early morning hours and at the time of her afternoon naps, more chair sensor firings during the night time and fewer during the day time, and an increase in activity of the bathroom PIR, fridge door contact sensor and electric usage sensor on the kettle during the night time. These changes seemed to correspond with an interpretation that Miss Evans was feeling increasingly unwell and restless in the period leading up to her hospitalisation and that her sleep pattern and overall well-being improved after her return from hospital. Subsequently, we sought a validation of our interpretation from the participant herself, and she confirmed our interpretation during the interview.

However, it also came to light during the interview that Miss Evans' medication on her return from hospital was stronger than the tablets she had been used to taking before. This had a direct impact on her behaviour in the evening and contributed to the altered pattern of sensor activity after her return from hospital, 'At night I'm more relaxed. I think the evening I can go quite drowsy and I'm pleased about that because I never used to be drowsy till I went to bed and then I couldn't sleep'. Other observed changes were clearly induced by the package of external care that had been prescribed for Miss Evans as part of her arrangements for hospital discharge, which represented an unwelcome curtailment of her domestic activities, 'They'd come at five to put me to bed, well I didn't really ... The evening ones worried me because I wanted a night. ... You see I'd no evening, you cut my evening out'.

This serves to emphasise the extreme difficulty that existed in interpreting the data obtained from LSM sensors without additional contextual information about what was actually happening in the home. In the example presented above, we assumed that the pattern of sensor firings after Miss Evans returned from hospital was more akin to a 'well-being pattern' than the pattern pre-hospitalisation, but it emerged that other factors such as medication and care services were also implicated in the changed pattern of observed sensor activity post-hospitalisation. Moreover, in a non-research setting, questions remain as to how to decide which pattern of sensor firings represents a 'norm' in the case of a particular individual. It is important to bear in mind that behavioural 'norms' may be fluid and may change over time, potentially influencing how to set the sensor parameters for raising alerts and who might be best placed to set these parameters for 'normal behaviour'.

LSM sensors are capable of spotting some changes in daily routines around the time of important life career events, but the results from this trial suggest that the interpretation of these changes requires a large amount of contextual information and the involvement of participants themselves. Much work remains to be done before it will become clear what is even meant in practice by a pattern in an individual's domestic activity, particularly where the person concerned leads a relatively routine-free lifestyle. Furthermore, the findings to date have highlighted technical and operational difficulties that need to be resolved before it will be possible to use LSM predictively.

Overall, the results from this small LSM trial suggest that the availability of contextual information about the events and everyday activities of participants is crucial, both at the stage of choosing appropriate LSM sensors and when attempting to provide a meaningful interpretation of their results. In order to 'make sense of sensors' alongside the data provided by the devices, one needs rich contextual information that is normally accumulated through social interactions between caregivers and care receivers, a two-way communication process that can best be described as a 'dialogue of care'.

Notes

1 The study was funded by the EPSRC EQUAL (grant GR/S 29058/01) and is part of a larger consortium that also included Barnsley Hospital NHS Foundation Trust, Dundee University, Imperial College London, a telecare supplier and a specialist housing and care provider. Plans of the participants' flats were prepared by David Thom of Stern Thom Fehler Architects Ltd.

8   The performativity of a volunteer-based telecare service

Darren Reed

Introduction

Telecare is a form of technology that directly affects people's lives. For many, the opportunity to support activities through technology is highly worthwhile. Those using telecare to support others are convinced of the benefits, yet these 'advocates' must survive in an atmosphere of administrative objectivity.

This chapter is based on the 'performative turn' in a range of disciplines including science and technology studies and social science more generally. It contrasts the performance of a telecare service as efficiency with its performativity through a conceptually based, layered analysis of the 'Befriending Scheme' run by the Community Resource Team (CRT) in Hackney, London. While the distinction between efficient performance and performativity is relatively clear, confusion is possible because of the use in some quarters of the term 'performativity' to refer to performance as efficiency. We will pursue this below with a discussion of Lyotard's (1984) use of the term.

What we are aiming for is an understanding of the performativity of age and technology, which recognises the narrative and interactional aspects of the support service in terms of identity, relationships and the interplay between technology and people in real instances of 'doing' telecare. We do this through a conceptual formulation that combines performative identity from Judith Butler and Ann Bastings and the temporal unfolding of human technology interaction from Andrew Pickering and Ian Hutchby, and biographical accounts of technology from the earlier work of the author.

This chapter also builds on an earlier study of telephone conferencing for older people from a combined human–computer interaction, conversation analytic perspective (e.g. Reed 2003, 2004; Reed & Monk 2004; Monk & Reed 2007). An understanding of the 'performativity of age and technology' offers a possibility for transformation such that telecare services might significantly improve the life experiences of clients through reinvigorated roles, relationships and self-understanding.

Background

The 'Befriending Scheme' is run by the CRT, part of Hackney Borough Council's support services. CRT has a number of aims and objectives, which include providing companionship for isolated older individuals through face-to-face and telephone contact, increasing participation in community life, providing valued information, and promoting healthy activity and independence. They are based on two principles: 'meeting the person, not just the need', and 'joining up and innovating' (Davis & Brown 2007: 4).

The team provides eight services in all: 'Home Visits', weekly visits by volunteers; 'Ring-a-Round', where one volunteer phones twenty or so clients for a brief chat; 'Card Service', when birthday, bereavement and other cards are sent to clients; 'Tele link up 2 U', a volunteer-facilitated teleconference-based group call; 'Wheelchair Service', in which volunteers who take immobile clients out on short visits; 'Social Gatherings', supported by specialist transport services; 'Two's Company', in which a volunteer accompanies a client on visits to the hospital, hairdresser, etc.; and the 'Counselling Support Service', which supports the emotional needs of volunteers.

The various service elements are targeted at those who will benefit from them. They are integrated, with each service supporting the others, and they comprise a deliberate strategic progression from isolation to social involvement and engagement with one element supporting another.

Currently, there are eighty volunteers and 211 clients. Table 8.1 shows the ages of the people involved as well as the relative weighting of each individual service area in December 2007 (at which point there were only 185 clients).

During the period of the fieldwork and study, the service was increasingly under financial pressure, to the extent that the teleconferencing groups were halved in frequency. It transpires that there is no ring-fenced budget for the telephone conference costs and, instead, funds are diverted from the general communication budget of the service. This chapter is seen as a means of qualifying the character of the telecare aspects in order to support its future development.

Table 8.1 Ages of the people involved as well as the relative weighting of each individual service area in December 2007

Services	Users	Gender		Diversity		Age range (years)	
Home visiting	45	Female	143	White	94	50–65	13
Ring-a-round	101	Male	42	Asian	6	66–75	38
Teleconferencing	28			Black	55	76–85	75
Two's company	4			Other	15	86+	47
Wheelchair	7			Not stated	7	*	
Card service	All			*			

* Some users may be in receipt of more than one service (Davis & Brown 2007).

Methodology

The research in the Befriending Scheme was part of a project at the University of York looking at technology-mediated communication as a means to support isolated and lonely older people. The Hackney work was a case study in the ethnographic stages of the research, alongside other group telephone support services provided through a not for profit company called Community Network in London. These services ranged from support for informal carers in the 'ring-around-carers' scheme to church service participation for housebound people.

The Hackney fieldwork comprised interviews with care professionals, participation and recording of teleconference calls and accompanied home visit interviews with clients of the service. The recordings were transcribed in line with a conversation analytic analysis (Atkinson & Heritage 1984) of the interaction. A number of other telephone calls of other groups were recorded, transcribed and analysed. In the second half of the project, insights gleaned from the ethnographic work were incorporated into lightweight experiments that manipulated features of the calls to see if the flow of the conversation could be affected, with the idea being that a more flowing conversation equates with a better experience of taking part (see Reed 2004; Monk & Reed 2007).

In the analysis that follows, we draw on three aspects of the data produced: care professionals' accounts of the assessment of the scheme; recordings of the Tele link up 2 U (henceforth 'link up' calls) and clients' experiential accounts of taking part. The analysis of the link up calls is necessarily brief but aims to indicate some examples of features that point up the performance of age categories in terms of membership category devices (MCDs), an analytic concept in conversation analysis.

We first need to introduce performativity in a brief conceptual section. We will develop the relevance of each aspect in the later discussion.

Conceptual foundations

Austin's linguistic theory

John Austin's (1962) distinction between the performative and the constative utterance underpins all the uses of the concept of performativity used here. A constative is defined as 'an utterance that asserts or states something that can be judged as true or false', while a performative is 'an utterance that performs an act or creates a state of affairs by the fact of its being uttered under appropriate or conventional circumstance' (Loxley 2006: 10). This distinction is the thread that joins together Pickering's understanding of technology development, Butler's understanding of identity and Basting's analysis of senior theatre groups in the USA. Austin's theory is also at the root of discourse analysis, through the work of Potter and Wetherell (1987), and provides for the conversation analytic rationale and practice. Lyotard's examination of knowledge also relies upon Austin's formulation, although in this case there is an alternative and distinct formulation of performativity.

Lyotard's performativity

A number of writers pursue a distinction made by Jean-François Lyotard (1984) between two forms of knowledge or language games, the scientific and the narrative (Dent & Whitehead 2002). In Lyotard's view, performativity signals the subordination and devaluation of the narrative form such that:

> The new discourse of truth about the world which emerges with scientific knowledge is one which brooks no challenge from narrative knowledge, for within this language game narrative knowledge becomes delegitimised as 'primitive, underdeveloped, backward … composed of opinions, customs, authority, prejudice, ideology'.
>
> Dent and Whitehead (2002: 8, quoting Lyotard 1984: 27)

Instead, what legitimises science and many other activities is the 'technological criterion' – the most efficient input/output ratio – or what Lyotard calls performativity (http://www.iep.utm.edu/l/Lyotard.htm). In these terms, performativity 'describes the endless search for effectiveness and efficiency in the contemporary "post-modern" society' (Kerfoot 2002). Professional standing, for example, has to be 'validated by scientific knowledge' and 'succumb to the pressure to be measured against so-called "objective criteria in scientific mode"' (Dent & Whitehead 2002: 8). According to Dent and Whitehead (2002: 8):

> Lyotard's use of performativity signals and defines the current obsession with 'efficiency' and the concern to 'objectively subject this efficiency to empiricist means and measures to test its worth'.

We could mount a critique of these thoughts by undermining the imperative of measuring performance. However, instead, we wish to incorporate this particular formulation of 'performativity' into a broader understanding of a continuum of performativity. At one end, this is measurable; at the other, it is not. Along the continuum, there are various moments where the measurable and the immeasurable, formal and informal, combine. An example we will see in a moment is where structured questionnaires are used to elicit experiential accounts from the scheme's participants. To enable our later discussion, we will call Lyotard's formulation 'efficiency-performativity'. In contrast, there are a number of authors who actively develop performativity in terms of the devalued narrative form of knowledge. We will label these approaches 'biographical-performativity'. To underline this description, we incorporate below work from biography and narrative approaches to gerontology.

Butler's performative identity

Judith Butler asserts that gender identity should be conceived as a performance, 'Gender ought not to be construed as a stable identity or locus of agency from which various acts follow; rather, gender is an identity tenuously constituted in time, instituted in an exterior space through a stylized repetition of acts' (Butler 1993: 179). Instead of a deliberate 'act', Butler (1993) sees gender as a 'reiterative and citational practice by which discourse produces the effects that it names'. Identity is achieved through the repetition of commonly held notions of appropriate behaviour and attitudes. It is 'cited', but at the same time seen as an authentic attribute in that 'its "citational nature" is "denied and concealed"' (Loxley 2006: 125). These ideas about the citational performance of identity have been taken into the study of age identity.

Age identity and performance

Ann Basting (1998) undertook an ethnographic study of senior theatre groups in the USA. Over a 2-year period, eight theatre groups' performances were studied through an ethnographic approach and analysed through a conceptually informed framework built on Butler's work.

In line with Butler, Basting notes that 'one is not born with a fixed identity, rather one congeals an identity through repeated performances or social practices across time' (ibid.: 7–8). Acceptance of this idea with regard to age identity is far easier than gender, which has to break away from the notion of naturalness. However, there is still an ingrained expectation that age identity is in some sense uniform, natural and inevitable. A large literature in gerontology has established a set of expectations around such notions as 'stages of life' and disengagement theory. In addition, the single focus on physical, cognitive and biological functioning tends to predominate and reinforce the naturalness of age.

Basting combines Butler with work of the theatrical performance theorist Richard Schechner (1985) to understand the possibility of the 'transformation' of age identity through theatre. This performance is transformative because it 'offers to both individuals and groups the chance to rebecome what they once were, or even, and most often, to rebecome what they never were but wish to have been or wish to become' (Basting 1998: 38). Butler sees transformation in the 'impossibility of exact repetition' (ibid.: 8), the 'ideal is never accomplished' (Butler 1990: 124) and identity is open to 'splittings, self-parody, [and] self-criticism' (ibid.: 146–47).

For Basting, in senior theatre activities, there is the possibility of creating 'a performance matrix in which meanings of old age can be questioned and potentially transformed' (ibid.: 9). In each of the various theatre groups, there are different levels of transformation based on how age identity is used and presented in the individual productions. One group, for example, parodies age-specific identities; another attempts to undermine expectations through gymnastic displays. Yet these are problematic because they retain an old/young distinction, rather than challenging received notions. Transformation is seen by Basting in performances that deepen the emotional insight of the audience, with empathy transgressing generational boundaries.

The same can be said about all instances of identity performance. As Loxley (2006) puts it '[performance] variance opens the door to political influence. It is possible for the identity to change over time with its "citationality" and "iterability" resulting in changes due to temporal drift or deliberate intervention' (ibid.: 147).

Pickering and the mangle of practice

Andrew Pickering (1995) engaged with scientific knowledge and technology development by championing a move from a 'representational' to a 'performative idiom' (ibid.: 5). Instead of understanding the world as composed of statements and descriptions that represent the world, wherein the prevailing question is the quality of these representations, he proposed a thoroughgoing change in perspective, which understands the temporal unfolding of science and technology practice as a matter of a 'dance of agencies' (ibid.: 102).

> One can start from the idea that the world is filled not, in the first instance, with facts and observations, but with agency. The world I want to say, is continually doing things, things that bear upon us not as observation statements upon disembodied intellects but as forces upon material beings. Think of the weather. Winds, storms, droughts, floods, heat and cold – all of these engage with our bodies as well as our minds, often in life-threatening ways … Much of everyday life, I would say, has this character of coping with material agency, agency that comes at us from outside the human realm and that cannot be reduced to anything within that realm.
>
> Pickering (1995: 6)

Through such a shift in perspective, a conception of human practice or agency is combined with a recognition of 'material agency'. At different points, the primary dynamic is provided by the machine, the material or the word configured in material terms; at others, it is the human action or interpretation. These processes unfold over time in a 'dance of agencies' (ibid.: 21–22) and, from a human perspective, appear as a form of interaction with the material world,

> the dance of agency, seen asymmetrically from the human end, thus takes the form of a *dialectic of resistance and accommodation*, where resistance denotes the failure to achieve an intended capture of agency in practice, and accommodation an active human strategy of response to resistance, which can include revisions to goals and intentions as well as to the material

form of the machine in question and to the human frame of gestures and social relations that surround it.

Pickering (1995: 22, emphasis added)

The dialectic of resistance and accommodation, Pickering calls the 'mangle of practice' (ibid.: xi), a term he picks because it indicates first the 'complexity of the "assemblage of multiple and heterogeneous elements" of social practice and culture, second it elicits a mental picture of the wooden rollers of the old fashioned device into which is fed the tangled clothes or sheets and out of which comes the squeezed, dried and compressed item'. Such a choice plays in two ways, it 'engenders a dynamic process wherein "to mangle" both references the processes of society, and also the processes of making sense and "straightening out" such complexity as knowledge' (ibid.: 22–23).

While Pickering's analysis is set at the level of scientific discovery (chapters 2, 3 and 4) and the implementation of technology in the engineering industry (chapter 5), he claims that the mangle is 'scale invariant' and can be seen at any level of analysis, ' ... at whatever level of magnification one interrogates history, one finds mangling. At the microlevel ... one finds micromangling; at the macrolevel, one finds macromangling' (ibid.: 234).

This scalability legitimises our layered analytic method, which sees the mangle at the level of assessment of the befriending service, in the interpretation and activities of its clients and in the conversational activity in telephone conference calls. In each instance, we can look to reveal and understand the temporal unfolding of 'resistance' and 'accommodation' in the story of the service. Added to Basting's conception of age identity, we can reveal instances of technologically afforded performances.

Biography of age and technology

Research into biography and ageing has revealed ageing 'from the inside' through an understanding of the centrality of people's discursively constructed narratives of life-course experiences (Birren *et al.* 1996; Ruth & Kenyon 1996). These insights extend from the idea that 'older people do not perceive meaning in aging itself; rather, they perceive meaning in being themselves in old age' (taken from Kaufman 1986: 6, quoted in Ruth & Kenyon 1996). Phillipson contrasts the biographical approach to ageing with those that concentrate on the 'technical' aspects of physical and mental function and contends that:

[b]y presenting ageing as a technical problem we have lost sight of the fact that it is 'biographical as well as biological'; that 'old age is an experience to be lived meaningfully and not only a problem of health and disease'.

Phillipson (1998: 23)

In human computer interaction (HCI), McCarthy and Wright (2004) seek to rediscover 'lived experience' through an understanding of the 'felt life' of technology. Drawing on the literary approach of Bhaktin and the pragmatic theory of Dewey, they define experience as 'the irreducible totality of people acting, sensing, thinking, feeling, and making meaning in a setting, including their perception and sensation of their own actions' (ibid.: 54). This rediscovery involves an understanding of the emotional, the sensual, the aesthetic, ongoing and open-ended incorporation and appropriation of technology into people's daily lives. It is essentially biographical in that it involves 'reflection' and the telling of stories about experience.

Analysis and discussion

In this section, we apply these conceptual insights to three aspects of the befriending scheme, conceived as three layers of performativity – the assessment of the scheme, interaction in the telephone conference calls and the experiential accounts of clients. In each instance, we identify aspects in terms of our conceptions of performativity. We see a progressive move away from 'efficient-performativity' as an appropriate framing and a move towards 'biographical-performativity'. We start by treating these elements separately by pointing up aspects that correspond to 'formal measures', 'identity' and the 'mangle of practice', but in each case these come together to form a correspondence of interests around the 'performativity of age and technology'. As we move towards it, we move increasingly away from efficient-performativity and the concomitant performance management ideas of prevailing ideals. The discussion that follows the analysis provides additional examples of performative layers. This deepens and summarises the total understanding of the performativity of age identity and technology in readiness for our comments in the conclusion.

Analysis 1: the assessment of the befriending scheme

A first point is that, by assessment, we focus on particular aspects of the service: the recruitment of volunteers, the referral and recruitment of clients and the monitoring of the relationship between client and volunteer. We could also include the training and review of volunteers and an overall understanding of the activity of the befriending scheme. Areas that we do not approach include the accreditation process by the Mentoring and Befriending Foundation (http://www.mandbf.org.uk/) and Hackney Borough Council's internal assessment of personnel.

Recruitment of volunteers

New volunteers are recruited through a variety of mechanisms, through local advertising in newspapers, doctor's surgeries and the like, as well as at social events such as an annual festival for older people and weekly social dance events.

Advertisements detail the qualities required, and each potential volunteer is sent an application form that asks questions about the person's experiences. These include their experience of volunteering in the past but crucially include their own personal experiences of life, such as whether they have cared for an elderly relative.

In an interview, potential volunteers are asked to imagine a scenario in which they are to spend an hour with a client. They then describe the sorts of things they would do and talk about.

> ROSE: you tend to get a feel by the way they respond to questions at interview ... you can hear the passion with the majority of them, and they will give you a scenario, or it might be I was brought up by my grand- mother or I looked after an older person who was a member of the family.
>
> Interview, 1 February 2008

An important aspect is the person's motivation:

> ROSE: in my own personal experience in terms of good and bad I tend to find irrelevant whether you've got an academic or you've got, you can read and write very well, I think the interest that comes across at the interview and how enthused somebody can be and how much knowledge they've got around your service that they've taken the time to read up about it.
>
> Interview, 1 February 2008

One professional puts the point simply as 'they must have the interests of people at heart' (Interview, 1 February 2008).

Many of the qualities looked for by service professionals in a future volun- teer are difficult to quantify. There is a strong sense of impressionistic and experiential insight being key judgement tools. It is in the way the person behaves and presents themselves – how they perform – in combination with their experience and expectations of the way interactions with clients will play out that decisions are made.

Recruitment of clients

Clients are referred by other care professionals, family and friends, but important questions are first asked about the level of need, based on daily experiences, and the appropriateness of the general befriending scheme. In short, the client is first matched with aspects of the service.

> ROSE: I'll give you an example, when Eric comes up for the assessment and through the questions that are asked, we look at, well do you attend a day centre? If you attend a day centre, how many days do you attend? And if for instance they say I go to the day centre twice a week and other

days I have meals on wheels or I have a carer that comes in to do my personal care seven days a week. Things like that or I've got regular contact with family and friends. They are not likely to get maybe the home visiting. Whereas someone who has little or no contact and perhaps maybe has personal care. They could have personal care seven days a week but the reality is those carers are limited by time as to how long they can stay with someone. They do their job and then they've gone. They could be left all day with no-one else to see them, or contact them on the telephone. So we would consider that person more suitable for home visiting.

Interview, 1 February 2008

It is not a simple matter to identify the needs of clients. They are buried under and in the details of daily life; their exposition is complex and involved. It requires common sense, such that an understanding of the 'reality of life' must be applied. There is also a strong sense of contingency in the reasoned outcome, based as it is on the best available knowledge. Outcomes, decisions, programmes of activities are similarly contingent, open to change as a result of new and better insight. In short, outcomes are never finalised. Such a logic and mentality leaves the door open to review and change at a later stage, either during the training and activities of volunteers or in the review and adaptation to the client's changing circumstances.

Ongoing monitoring of the volunteer

Once a volunteer is chosen, they go through a period of training and are invited into formal assessment interviews after prescribed periods: initially after 6 weeks, then 6 months and after that every 12 months. In addition to these specified points, the training period is an opportunity for unofficial assessment and is a springboard for continued unofficial monitoring. The care professional who carries out the training is also the trained counsellor; this twin role of training and support of the volunteers provides for a personal interaction centred upon the volunteer's motivation and needs. It is also a continual conduit back to the remaining care professionals.

Monitoring the relationship between client and volunteer

Successful volunteer applicants are matched with clients. Much of the ongoing assessment revolves around this relationship such that conversations with volunteers and clients at defined times are oriented to how they interact, whether this results in benefits for the client and whether the relationship should continue.

A key component of this monitoring is the application of a standardised questionnaire in a home visit by one of the care professionals. Its actual utility is in the way it prompts accounts of the client's experiences of the service and the volunteer.

ROSE: But it's the way you pose questions, because you get a feel, and everything else that comes with it, and there's a comments box so that we can fill in, and see what the client says. It's very hard to put into numbers, that's really informative that information. The questions are 'do you find the service satisfactory, not satisfactory, very satisfactory for instance'.

Interview, 1 February 2008

The questions 'do you want the service to continue' and 'do you want the same person to provide the service' are deliberate prompts for personal accounts of the ongoing relationship between client and volunteer.

What characterises this assessment activity is the combination of formal and informal activities and measures seen most clearly in the professional's use of the questionnaire to prompt deeper insight. Applying our conceptual model, we can detect a temporal dialectical unfolding in the imposition of formal questions and the resistance and accommodation to them through experiential accounts of the client. The formal questionnaire becomes the mechanism or material agency that provokes these performative accounts.

Taken together, these various assessment activities amount to a continual, open-ended and unfinished process. We might say that they amount to a 'network of mundane assessment' where this network involves people and techniques in formal and informal interactions. At different points, these processes coalesce to form decisions to employ recruits or accept clients, but they immediately open out again into ambiguity and complexity. Assessment re-emerges as a 'matter for conversation', reiteration and review.

Strategies of performativity

Ultimately, the assessment of the befriending scheme rests on a specific outcome, the reduction of social isolation of its clients. As we have seen above, at various points, questions about levels of loneliness and isolation are incorporated into the interaction with clients. Overarching these targeted measures is a deliberate strategy of increased involvement, achieved through the different affordances of the services. We can detail this strategy by considering the progression of 'client career' (Brink 1986).

Another performative layer can be seen in the scheme's strategy for combating social isolation. Clients are referred to the service by professionals and non-professionals. For example, they may have had a period of hospitalisation or may have fallen in their homes and been referred by social services. A visit by one of the three befriending officers determines their needs and abilities (such as level of mobility, emotional state and communicative need). A typical progression would then be to enrol them in the ring-around service and card service. In this way, an isolated individual has regular contact and begins to acclimatise to social interaction. From this, they may be invited to take part in a teleconference group, which meets once every 2 weeks. From here, they are encouraged to attend social gatherings, with the help of the specialised transport service and wheelchair service. At each point, they come into contact with increasing numbers of volunteers and clients, which taps directly into the play of agencies and various affordances (technological and human) of the befriending service. It also expresses the play of resistance and accommodation mentioned by Pickering.

The strategy also plays out naturally in the calls themselves through the dynamics of socialisation in the telephone conference calls and the motivations of participants to form welcoming and inclusive groups.

By way of example, during one of the calls recorded for the research, a single male, who was also interviewed in person by the researcher, is in conversation with four females and a befriending officer, Eric. The group has been meeting for some months, and Derek has been part of the service for 4 years. In that time, he has never met any of the other clients in person. The atmosphere is playful, and the participants feel they can speak freely and openly as friends even though they have never met the man.

S: Eric, tell Derek to come here, he'd love it here
E: yeah
S: Eric, tell, tell him
E: yeah it's a lovely place, you'd love it
S: you'd like it here, you'd settle in here
D: I've been in a couple of times and I know how lovely it is
S: Eric tell Derek about my flat
E: Cyril if you go there, you will love it
S: he can come round if he wants to
E: yeah
S: he'd love it ere
E: yeah
...
S: we have parties, we have parties there
D: I'll tell you what we've got there Cyril we've got a very nice doctor (.) doctor Redin
S: yeah, I've got doctor Redin as my doctor
D: He's a friend of mine, he's lovely

                    Simplified transcript (link up call, 22 July 2002)

This is one simple example where the tendency of the group is to encourage increased involvement and, in this case, a move to physical co-location. The official strategy and overall aims of the service combine with the motivations of the clients. The performativity of the strategy plays out at both the level of progressive service–client matching and in the mundane everyday interaction of the calls.

The reason for adding this example is again to stress the combination of formal and informal interaction. It is difficult to see how an efficiency notion of performativity could adequately characterise these combined strategies, not least because they are uncoordinated and bear little relation to one another. Not only is it difficult to quantify social isolation, but it would be an impaired mode of assessment that did not incorporate the interpersonal processes.

Another way to understand the performativity is at the level of an individual telephone conference. We can approach this in two ways, in Pickering's terms as the temporal play of agencies, and also in Butler and Basting's understanding of identity.

Analysis 2: a close reading of teleconference interaction

In the following section, we undertake a close reading of the actual speech in the teleconferencing calls. We do this from a conversation analytic perspective. Austin's distinction between the performative and the constative is at the basis of certain forms of discourse analysis, particularly Loughborough University's Discourse and Rhetoric Group (DARG) (of which the author was a member). Talk-in-interaction in conversation analysis has a performative quality, and many of the empirical findings and conceptions of conversation analysis can be applied to close readings of the performance of identity (Antaki 1998) and technology interaction (Reed & Ashmore 2000; Reed 2001).

A characteristic feature of conversation analysis is a keen attention to the 'sequential' nature of interaction. This has been called the 'CA analytic mentality' by Schenkein (1978). We incorporate this mentality into a description of a single telephone conference call, as a means to orient the reader to a sequential reading of the conversation.

Telephone as material agency

As a starting point, we can note that telephone calls have 'clearly demarcated beginnings and endings', and the beginnings and endings of telephone calls are 'distinctive interactional events' that, among other things, allow people to 'manage intimacy at a distance' (Hutchby 2001: 89).

First, a description of the progression of a typical conference call: at a pre-booked time, an operator from Community Network telephones a series of numbers. Typically, the first person to be contacted is the volunteer 'facilitator'; however, if this person fails to answer, then the next person on the participant list is contacted. Once contacted, the first person is 'placed in the call' by themselves. They move from talking to the operator to sitting holding the telephone with no noise in the handset. The operator then contacts the next person on the list, perhaps returning to the facilitator if necessary. Again, a conversation ensues between operator and participant and, at the end of this interaction, the operator 'announces' the person to the single person in the call. The time between the first and second participant can be seconds or minutes depending on the availability of the 'next' participants. The single individual is met with the announcement 'hello Doris, I have Derek for you'. A greeting ensues between Doris and Derek. Some moments later, the operator returns and announces a new participant. If the facilitator is present, the new person is introduced to them; if not, the new person is introduced to the membership as a whole: 'hello everyone, I've got Margaret for you'. The routine continues until all the participants have been introduced. At times, when a participant is not immediately available, they may be contacted 10 minutes into the call. If the conversation is flowing, the operator can find it difficult to make themselves heard and may try to stop the conversation.

If we think in terms of the 'stabilisation' of a group call, incorporating language from the social construction of technology and used by Pickering to talk about large-scale technology implementations, we can say that the process starts with technological agency, the ringing telephone summoning the first person to participate (Schegloff 1977 – see later), and ends with the last person being successfully introduced into the call. Of course, beyond this initial stabilisation of call participation is the ensuing group conversation. If instead we talk about the 'stabilisation' of a group conversation, the plain fact is that it may never happen during a single call; it may be that it never happens that all the participants share the conversational floor and feel empowered to take part. A facilitator interviewed for the study states that sometimes it simply does not happen. People feel unable to take part, distanced from the other participants, sitting in their own home. The material agency of the telephone and its remote position impedes their participation. Indeed, some participants, such as Derek mentioned earlier, actively take a back seat role. They prefer to listen rather than talk. In this sense then, the affordance of the group telephone call allows for a particular behaviour. One participant likened listening to the group conference call as reminiscent of the possibilities afforded by the 'party line' system of telephone provision. Here, a single telephone line was shared by a number of families. It was a guilty secret that some evenings were spent listening to other people's calls!

Identity and interaction in the telephone conference

Pirjo Nikander (2000, 2002) incorporates the CA notion of membership categorisation devices (MCDs) (Silverman, 1998) into her analysis of age identity in talk-in-interaction. Nikander's work also serves here as an introduction to discursive approaches to age identity (see also Jones 2006 and 'discursive gerontology').

Quoting Edwards (1991), Nikander notes that 'Discursive research ... treats talk and texts not as representations of pre-formed cognitions ... but as forms of social action. Categorisation is *something we do*, in talk, in order to accomplish social actions (persuasion, blamings, denials, refutations, accusations etc.)' (p. 517, emphasis in original). This positions age categories as a form of performative action, rather than cognitive or biological representation.

Such an approach breaks free from 'the notion of age as mere unproblematic background variable' (p. 4), and her task is to 'produce empirically grounded observations on the communicative practices through which age identity and age categories are applied, modified, and challenged in talk, and to show the kinds of interactional business that is achieved through its definition and re-formulation'. She wishes to 'show how age categories function as flexible sense-making resources' (p. 5, old vs. little girls).

MCDs and flow in telephone conferences

We should re-emphasise the unfamiliar nature of talking on the telephone in groups. On each occasion, participation is not immediately fluid. There is a great deal of talk about who is present and the like. Talk 'about' talking on the telephone in groups is a repeated conversational item.

The 'communicative affordances' of the telephone set up particular technology-oriented identities. These 'novel categorial identities', as Hutchby (2001) calls them, comprise 'caller', 'called' and 'answerer' (ibid.: 101). These identities ratify and constrain behaviour, such that it is typically the 'caller' who introduces conversational topics, at least initially in the form of 'reasons for call'. Call opening implies a particular power relationship that Hopper calls 'caller hegemony' (1992).

It is not unusual for conversations to include talk about age and age identity. The following are two instances in separate calls of when age identity, specifically the use of the category 'girls', becomes a matter of hilarity.

R: okay girls so now we can start our chat
A: girls (.) girls (.) a wish (.) a wish
D: [those were] the days
R: yeah well ner mind never mind soo any of you goin on holidee

Link up call, 25 July 2002

L: right well there's just the three of us then girls
R: ah [he he he he]he he he
D: [he he he he]
R: girls lovely
L: so what did you do over the weekend, if we start off with you rose.(.) did you do anything exciting

Link up call, 25 July 2002

Without going too deep into the interaction taking place in this second instance, up to this point in the call, participants had been quiet and there had been no group chat. The comment 'girls lovely' is met with laughter by the remaining group members, who then participate from this point onwards as a group. The instantiation of age identity has a direct impact upon the conversational flow and the agency of the participants.

In other writing, the author conceives a 'measure of flow' in the telephone conferences, as the rate of conversational participation (see Reed 2004; Monk

& Reed 2007) in combination with an analysis of the actual content of the interaction. An understanding of a 'good' conversation in terms of 'flow' is little use without knowing the nature of the interaction. Participants may be arguing, for example. In other words, measurement alone cannot fully characterise human interaction, and conversation is not something that can be captured by notions of efficiency.

Technology affordance and age identity behaviour

Basting (1998) expresses reservations about some senior theatre events that present age identity in particular ways. Likewise, it is possible to approach the activity of taking part in a telephone conference as re-establishing particular age identities. An example here is a product of all telephone calls, the opening 'how are you' turn-taking routine. It has been shown that such 'openings' have a particular 'canonical' character (Table 8.2).

In a telephone conference, there are repeated 'openings' as each person is introduced into a conversation. Time after time, a new person is greeted and asked how they are. What is remarkable is that, on virtually each occasion, the response is not a typical or nominal greeting 'second' (Hutchby & Wooffitt 1998) such as 'fine, how are you', but instead an account of how the person is. Betty, one of the volunteer facilitators, describes it this way: 'The first thing you ask is how are you, all that jazz. There's not one of us without an ache or pain so that takes some time' (Interview, January 2003). What this means for the telephone conferences in the befriending scheme is that the 'introductions' are extended and often involve a good deal of talk about health and other issues before the 'chat' proper starts.

Let us be clear, these comments are in no way a criticism of those taking part in the calls; however, the particular material agency and affordances of the telephone conference technologies instantiate repeated call openings. If, for example, all the people were to meet in person in a group, the possibility of

Table 8.2 Examples of the particular 'canonical' character of telephone 'openings'

Example telephone opening	Sequence elements
(Telephone ring)	
R: Hello	Summons/answer
C: Hello Ida?	
R: Yeah	Identification/recognition
C: Hi, =This is Carla	Greetings
R: Hi Carla.	Initial enquiries or 'how are you'
C: How are you.	
R: Okay:.	
C: Good.=	
R: =How about you.	
C: Fine. Don wants to know....	Caller's move to first topic

Note: Developed from Schegloff (1977).

each person taking this conversational opportunity might well be curtailed. It is the particular play of agencies here that encourages such activities. The 'citation' of a typical age-related conversational behaviour is enhanced because of the particular material agencies in play.

By way of balancing out what might be seen to be a negative take on the affordances of the telephone conference calls, another affordance of the group telephone call is the ability to listen to other people speaking. A facilitator, Betty, whose job it is to ensure that people have equal opportunity to talk in the call, recognises that 'some people like to just listen'. Elsie, a participant, when asked if it's difficult to speak on the calls, says 'sometime, but it passes the time anyway whoever is talking, dohnit' (Interview, January 2003). Another listener likened the ability to listen to childhood experiences of 'party line' telephone facilities, where a number of families would share a single telephone line. Listening to other people's calls was a form of entertainment which, while frowned upon, was surely the source of a great deal of enjoyment, she says.

These comments about technology-afforded identity work are clear examples of the performativity of age and technology.

Analysis 3: technology as biography and lived experience

Before we consider the performativity of age and technology more broadly, there is one other level of performativity revealed in the interviews with befriending scheme clients. Here we most fully see biographical-performativity in play in the stories people tell about their lived experience of the scheme and their 'resistance' to and 'accommodation' of various technologies in their life.

Derek, mentioned earlier, is visually impaired. Because he can care for himself, he gets few visits from support services such as meals on wheels or an attending care worker. He has a small portable television set, which he has switched on, but cannot see. He says that he finds the voices on the television comforting.

As with many of those interviewed, Derek initially found the idea of a teleconference mysterious and was nervous about taking part. However, he has become entirely comfortable talking and listening to other people. When asked why this was, he says, 'In my mind I imagine all the others in the same room', and then he conceives his interaction with a telephone conference in terms of his experiences of listening to the radio and television. He often speaks to the radio and television, he says, making comments about the content, and the telephone call is much like this. He rarely gets to speak anyway, he says, because the group is made up mainly of women (Interview, January 2003).

Doris is an educated women who lives in a large house by herself. She feels independent and has resisted selling her house and moving into smaller or shared accommodation. She is very active in her church, supporting and advising others. She fell recently and was found by her son. Social services had provided her with a fall pendant that she could wear around her neck in case it happened again, but she refuses to use it. Instead, she carries her DECT phone with her wherever she goes. Her son has programmed in his mobile number on quick dial and so she feels that, if she were to fall again, she could reach him immediately.

In the cases of both Derek and Doris, the technology, while initially a matter of resistance, has been accommodated into their own understandings of themselves and others. The dance of material agencies has played out such that each has incorporated and appropriated the telephone into their life.

Other participants speak of making the teleconference a meaningful event in their daily lives. One person makes a cup of tea before the call and readies herself in her favourite chair. Another has moved from being a recipient of the service to becoming a volunteer herself.

Discussion

Performance, efficiency and biography

There is a distinction to be had between business notions of 'performance' (Dent 2002) – what we have termed 'efficiency-performativity' – and health care ideas of 'assessment' (Heath & Watson 2005). The latter is far more concerned with the everyday, the qualitative and the experiential. Yet while we might expect such notions of assessment to have reached schemes such as that in Hackney, the interviews indicate that professionals in the befriending scheme understand 'proper' assessment in terms of ratings and measurements. At the same time, many of their accounts attach great value to the additional conversations and chats they have with colleagues, volunteers and clients. This emphasis is reminiscent in science and technology studies of two forms of discourse around science, the empiricist and the contingent repertoire. Drawing on Gilbert and Mulkay's (1984) work, Kevin Burchell (2007) notes the strategic *performativity* of the two repertoires in scientists' talk about themselves as grounded in empirical truth and others (scientists and non-scientists) mired in interpersonal and contextual complexity.

With the assessment of the befriending scheme, it is easy to see how performance measures, created and revealed in measurable answers, are prioritised as 'grounded' evidence, while interpersonal and contextual matters are mere background. Lyotard's technological criterion of efficiency in science pervades the befriending scheme's public presentation of itself in reports, and its own understanding of itself, but his performativity-as-efficiency is at the same time overwhelmed by the business at hand, which is shot through with contingent, relational and contextual knowledge.

In one sense, this chapter argues for a move towards biographical methods through its account of performativity, which is understood as a tuning or redefinition of the central term of performance. Yet, at the same time, we have seen moments when the contingent repertoire of experiential accounts relies wholeheartedly on empirical mechanisms.

The befriending scheme as a mangle of practice

The befriending scheme is a mangle of practice working at different scales or levels of abstraction. In general terms, we can see various material aspects of the world impacting upon the befriending service. Material agency is seen in geographical distance, the inability to leave the home, the broken hip, the failing eyesight and hearing. Resistance and accommodation occur in the everyday lives and behaviour of clients, volunteers and service professional. Returning to the issue of service assessment in the Hackney Befriending Scheme, the 'straightening out' of assessment occurs in and through complex processes and relationships. The 'service' as a unified whole is a combination of people, activity and interactions; recruitment is an issue of tuning; review is a dance of agencies.

Our comment above on assessment could be seen as revealing one layer of analysis. The informal assessments that interweave the more formal mechanisms reveal a form of behaviour and performance. Taken as material narratives, these mechanisms could be seen to 'dance' as in Pickering's description with those of the informal kind. Further, the informal feedback aspects that are carried out by telephone could be seen to require, rely and depend upon the relationships between human behaviour and technological affordance (Hutchby 2001).

We see in the care professional's accounts of the recruitment of the volunteers the unspoken requirement that they *perform* the role of volunteer by exhibiting and citing particular qualities, interests and future behaviour. The potential client is couched in the discourse of 'needs' and of the matching of these needs to the services provided. We get a sense of performativity in the logic of matching, through comparisons of everyday experiences and the potential intermingling of service elements to effect a particular outcome of inclusion, activity and wholeness, and ultimately of well-being. The befriending scheme's maxim of 'meet the person, not just the need' and the one it applies to the volunteer of 'having the interests of the people at heart' reinforce the biographical, emotional and motivational.

The reasoning employed in the interview about recruitment is itself a form of performance. It 'cites' the importance of an understandable and repeatable set of criteria as key to good judgement, but indicates at the same time the possibility of a mass of external, undefinable issues and instances that might affect such apparently understood processes of knowledge making. The net result is a 'straightening out' of these processes through the mangling of known (empirical) and unknown (contingent) elements in the process of the interview itself. Resulting in something like a 'weight of experience' acceptance, that they know what they are doing and are able to do this repeatedly over time.

The 'network of mundane assessment' is in part made possible by what is called in STS the various 'assemblages' of technology (Sismondo 2003) and their existing presence and meanings in people's lives. So, for example, without the telephone already installed in the client's home, many of the most vital aspects of the befriending scheme would not be possible. Taking this point further, without the acceptance of the telephone as a means to engender and sustain personal relationships, the telephone could not play this role of support. A simple example of how the telephone characterises and affords particularly valuable aspects of the service is in the way it allows for active feedback to housebound people. Similarly, the 'ring-around' calls are opportunities for informal information exchange (such as social aspects of the service) and news gathering. Communication with the centre is again afforded by the technology.

In different ways, when we examine the detail of the telephone conferences, whether that is the sequential unfolding of the technologically afforded interaction or the content of the actual conversation, we see the intermingling of technology and people. While particular identity-based behaviours are afforded participants, it is not the case that they are predetermined or inevitable. Drawing back to the earlier work by Basting, we might ask whether these technology–human relations promote 'transformation'. Or do they simply provide opportunity for the citing of age identity markers. We can perhaps see instances in which the brevity of the link up calls combined with the technological affordances conspire to merely reiterate the gross level of age identity. Butler would have it that transformation is an inevitable consequence of interaction, and therefore simply affording interaction is enough to bring about change in people's sense of self. With increased interaction comes the possibility for reflection, re-evaluation and transgressive iteration.

What is clear is that questions such as these are only possible with a 'biographical-performativity' approach to assessment. Only when we take seriously the effect that technology can have on a person's sense of self, their lived experience, can we fully unearth the value of such telecare initiatives.

Conclusion: performativity of age and technology in telecare services

Our various analytic examples have drawn upon a conceptual basis in linguistics, identity and technology studies. We have attempted to give examples that move towards an integration of a 'biographical-performativity' into an understanding of a telecare service. Such a move does not reject existing performance measure activities or formal mechanisms, but instead understands their application as part of the overall performativity of the service. The result is the possibility for a deep understanding of the way the telecare service, understood as a collection of people and technologies, affects older people's lives. Rather than presenting a systematic method, we hope the examples encourage future analysis by pointing the way to a performativity of age and technology.

9 From have nots to watchdogs

Understanding Internet health communication behaviors of online senior citizens

Sally J. McMillan, Elizabeth Johnson Avery and Wendy Macias

Introduction

Older Americans are often framed as 'have nots' in a world where 'born digital' young people rule everything from programming the video cassette recorder (VCR) to posting videos on YouTube (Fox & Madden 2005; Willis 2006). But the older population is not mired in an analog era. The Pew Internet and American Life Project reports that Internet use is growing rapidly among older populations (Fox & Madden 2005). Among those who are just entering their senior years, many are Internet users: 68 per cent of those aged 55–59 and 55 per cent of those aged 60–64. More than half of Americans aged 65–69 (57 per cent) report that they are online. The drop in use seems to begin at age 70 with only 27 per cent of those aged 70–75 using the Internet. Among the oldest Americans (age 75+), 17 per cent are Internet users (Fox & Madden 2005). It is possible that people who now use the Internet at work will continue to be Internet users even when their work years have ended. This suggests a possible growth in adoption among older seniors in the near future; particularly as baby boomers age over the next decade, the proportion of seniors using the Internet will continue its rapid growth (Rideout et al. 2005).

Older adults are among the heaviest users of the Internet for health-related information (Fox & Rainie 2002; Holstein & Lundberg 2003; Macias & McMillan 2008). About 70 per cent of online seniors report using the Internet for health information (Fox & Fallows 2003). Perhaps one motivation for the heavy use is the perceived trustworthiness of online health information; a Kaiser Family Foundation survey revealed that, for adults aged 50–64, the Internet is considered a more trustworthy source of health information than any traditional mass medium other than books. This trust placed in online health information issues an important warning to practitioners and scholars, as we must stress to senior audiences the importance of filtering and checking information sources (Rideout et al. 2005).

Researchers have examined ways to make health-related websites more accessible to older adults (Marwick 1999; Cohen 2001; Vanderheiden & Iacona 2001; Flynn et al. 2006) and have reported on the development of training programs that had a positive impact on seniors' use of online health information (Morrell 2002; Kaufman & Rockoff 2006). One example of a successful training program was a joint-sponsored project to 'train trainers' of senior citizens across the USA on how to use the Internet for health information. The project was designed to give older adults better access to valuable health information on the Internet and to enable them to evaluate and share this information. This training had a positive effect on the confidence of seniors who used the Internet for health information as well and also shared this health information with family and friends (Mehnert & Gardner 1998). However, relatively few scholarly studies have probed for in-depth understanding of seniors' use of the Internet for health information (Macias & McMillan 2008).

The primary purpose of this study is to gain insight into the older Americans who are already using the Internet. In particular, how do they view this digital environment as a resource for health information? Studying these Internet-active seniors is important because they represent a first wave of future health trends. Studies have shown that the baby boom generation is expected to place new burdens on the health care system as members of that population age (Llewellyn *et al.* 2004). But this generation that was born in the decades immediately following World War II is also far more technologically savvy than earlier generations (Willis 2006). Thus, by studying current online seniors, as well as some of the older members of the baby boom generation, we can begin to detect future patterns in the uses of technology for health information seeking. Qualitative methods are particularly useful because such methods allow for depth of insight to emerge from participants in a way that the many quantitative studies of online health information seeking (Flynn *et al.* 2006; Fox 2006; Hesse *et al.* 2006) cannot.

This study uses a grounded theory approach to address the phenomenon of senior citizens' use of online health information (Corbin & Strauss 1990; Strauss & Corbin 1990). This approach allows the theory to emerge from the insights provided by participants rather than imposing pre-existing theoretical perspectives from the literature.

Method

Data were collected via an online survey that was administered in late summer 2006. The sample for this study was selected from an online panel administered at the University of Texas at Austin.[1] Therefore, a purposive sample was used. The panel comprised 55 per cent women and 45 per cent men with varied educational backgrounds (13 per cent high school, 24 per cent some college, 32 per cent college graduate and about 26 per cent post-baccalaureate degree).

The key recruitment criterion for respondents was that they must be aged 55 or older. We used this lower limit on age because it is the age by which some baby boomers might be starting to retire (22.0 per cent of respondents aged 55–59 reported that they have retired and another 11.5 per cent have dropped to part-time work). We wanted to capture those boomers to begin to understand the impact they might have on future trends in online health communications. Even though some of the younger members of the study might not consider themselves 'seniors', we have used that term throughout for convenience.

Procedure

The panel members were emailed an invitation to participate in early August 2006 and a reminder was sent out a week later. The survey was closed in late August.

A probabilistic method was used to award ten respondents a cash prize for incentives. Those who responded to the initial email had a chance to win one US$100 grand prize, two US$75 second place prizes or two US$50 third place prizes. After a reminder email was sent, additional prizes of the same amount and quantity were offered. The recipients were notified and paid their prize amount by the survey panel administrators after the survey was completed.

A total of 1,530 invitations were sent and 237 emails were returned as undeliverable (1,293 is the baseline). A total of 424 individuals responded, resulting in a valid response rate of 32.8 per cent. This response rate resulted in a sample that is fairly representative of the panel.

Sample

The sample skewed slightly toward women (55.2 per cent), but men were also well represented (44.8 per cent), similar to the panel composition. Average age of respondents was 61.34 years with a range of 55–90 years. The participants were most likely to identify themselves as white (94.3 per cent), but there were a few minority participants (Hispanic 3.1 per cent, black 2.1 per cent, native American 1.7 per cent, and Asian 0.7 per cent). Because the survey was conducted online, it drew only from seniors who are Internet users. Looking at these individuals, who in many cases may be early adopters (Rogers 1995) of technology, can suggest the future evolution of online health information behaviors as even more seniors go online in the future.

Participants were generally well educated, even more so than the panel from which the respondents were drawn. All but 12 per cent had at least some college education; 52.2 per cent had earned at least a bachelor's degree and 28.8 per cent had earned a post-baccalaureate degree. Slightly more than a third (36.6 per cent) were retired while about a quarter (28.3 per cent) reported that they were still working full time. The remaining participants blended part-time work with child/grandchild/parent care and/or self-employment. The mode for household income range was US$65,000–$79,999, but income range was wide with about 8 per cent reporting that they earn less than US$20,000 annually and about 14 per cent reporting income of US$125,000 or more. On average, respondents seemed to be in fairly good health with a mean of 3.57 (scale of 1–5 with 5 being stronger agreement) in response to the statement: 'compared to others my age, I think I am in better health' (range 1–5, SD 1.219). A separate full report on all survey data provides more detail on links between demographic and socioeconomic factors and use of the Internet for health information (McMillan & Macias, forthcoming).

Generally, respondents seem to be fairly computer savvy with 84.4 per cent indicating that they have used a computer for 6 or more years and 80.5 per cent indicating that they have been using the Internet for 6 or more years. Only about 1 per cent of the respondents were 'newbies' to either the computer or the Internet, indicating that they had used these technologies for less than a year. The most common location for Internet access was the participants' home with 97.9 per cent indicating that they sometimes or often access the Internet at home. The second most common Internet access point was work with 40.9 per cent reporting that they sometimes or often go online at work.

For the purpose of the current study, a single question was the basis for analysis: 'We'd like any general feedback from you on the Internet, health care issues for seniors, and/or this survey. Please type as much as you would like in the space below.' A total of 357 (84.2 per cent) of the participants provided substantive (often multiparagraph) answers to this question. Those answers are analyzed to address the core question: how do online older Americans view the digital environment of the Internet as a resource for health information?

Two researchers used an approach described by Corbin and Strauss (Corbin & Strauss 1990; Strauss & Corbin 1990) to analyze data gathered from this open-ended survey question. This began with open coding that identified each separate topic introduced by participants in their response to the open-ended survey question. First, coders eliminated 'generic' comments about the survey itself (e.g., 'an interesting survey') so that the focus would remain on the primary research question. A total of 354 separate responses on topics related to the research question were identified. The second stage was what Corbin and Strauss call 'axial coding.' In this stage, both researchers individually analyzed all responses identified in open coding and attempted to group them into related categories. Each identified eight primary topic areas. While there were some slight differences in how they defined those categories, the researchers were able to come to agreement on the following eight primary topic areas: invaluable resource, fear of misinformation, public policy and governance, prescription drugs, deferment to doctors, actively managing their own health, social/lifestyle issues, and technological/information savvy. In the final stage of 'selective coding,' the researchers identified three overarching themes that cut across all the data: empowerment, personal and professional communities, and watchdogs and peer assumptions. A third researcher who was familiar with the topic, but who had not engaged in the coding process, reviewed the axial and selective coding and found no substantial problems with the way that the data were organized.

Axial coding categories

The axial coding categories represent a topical grouping of the ideas expressed by study participants in their open-ended responses to the question about

Internet use and health care. Each of the eight topics is introduced briefly and illustrated with representative quotes from study participants. Pseudonyms and participant age are provided for each quote.

Invaluable resource

A very common response from participants was that they had found the Internet to be an invaluable source of information for health as well as other topics. Often, these responses contrasted the Internet with other, non-digital sources of information.

> Excellent source for initial research and investigation. Much more reliable than medical reference books which are always going to be somewhat out-of date.
>
> Jane, 63

Participants also sometimes noted that the Internet was a two-edged sword when they were looking for specific information. Some found that they could get very detailed information on very specific topics, while others felt the need for information that was more specifically targeted toward their needs:

> I am pleased to find information on medicines, diseases, locations of doctors etc., but wish there were more information specifically for seniors.
>
> Ann, 61

An interesting subset of the responses focuses on the level of detail that is available in online resources. Most respondents were pleased to be able to go beyond the 'basic' information they could find at other sources.

> The internet has added a new dimension to my life. Anything can be accessed. I can find answers to all my questions; whether large or small. I go straight to the internet to find out what lab results mean, what words in a report mean, other opinions on various diseases or procedures I am interested in.
>
> Sam, 59

> I have found a lot of information on various medical issues on the internet. I can spend as much time as I want and don't feel pressured as I sometimes do when I try to get questions answered at the clinic.
>
> Betty, 61

Several respondents also noted that the Internet gave them more access to alternative information that is not available through the mainstream medical community.

> I have found very clear and helpful alternative advice. Even though every person beside me in my family is a physician, I use the internet for

perspective, context, and to assure me I can wait and rethink the problem before beginning a course of drugs.

> Joan, 61

Finally, many participants offered generic statements indicating that they felt much online health information is of high quality.

> I have found sites like the 'Merck Manual' quite helpful with up-to-date information on medical diagnoses and courses of treatment.
>
> Ron, 64

Fear of misinformation

As noted above, many respondents reported finding good information online. But many also expressed concerns about information quality. While many found the Internet to be a superior source of information, others preferred more traditional communication mechanisms.

> I really prefer 'hardcopy' so that I can pick the information up again and again. Sometimes I pass on information to family and friends (usually from doctor's newsletter); e.g., the use of vitamin B-6 (last week to a friend who has carpal tunnel syndrome).
>
> Dianna, 58

Others indicated that they might start an information search on the Internet, but proceed from there with caution – checking other resources as available.

> In general, the value of having the internet as a source to check medications, diseases, syndromes and just general information is high. It should always be used with caution, and as an adjunct to other medical systems and sources.
>
> Ruth, 56

However, this practice may be more of the exception than the rule. Most seniors fail to check the source of online health information. A recent study found that less than one in five seniors reports checking the source of information most of the time; more than half of them reported 'never' or 'hardly ever' checking sources (Rideout *et al.* 2005). The disturbing implications of seniors who use but do not filter this information indicate that preventing a false sense of security with the information is a necessary part of online training for senior adults using online health information.

Many respondents addressed the challenges of separating out good information from misinformation online.

> There is a lot of information out on the internet related to health issues. The problem is that verifying its accuracy and relevance is difficult, even for

those of us with a healthcare background. Finding alternative solutions to a problem is the biggest source of misinformation, it seems to me. If I have arthritis and look for information, there is some accurate information on medications, some frighteningly inaccurate information on medications, and contradictory information on alternative ways of easing arthritis pain.

Trish, 60

Respondents also provided some insights into strategies that they use for distinguishing between misinformation and helpful health information. These strategies often focused on selecting appropriate domains for information gathering.

The internet is a really good source for health information if you choose your source sites wisely. There are a number of sites with misinformation. If you stick to hospital, research centers and government sites, the information is very good.

Amy, 75

Concerns about misinformation extended to specific types and sources of online communication, with participants often addressing the potential bias that certain individuals and organizations might bring to online communication.

In general I think the internet is a good source of information but desperate people could be easily led astray; also I think chat and discussion boards on this type of thing lend themselves to those with an axe to grind. Or, rather, those who have had problems with surgery/chemotherapy/treatments/doctors, rather than those who have had a good outcome and moved on. It is good to KNOW about the problems, but you must be aware you're probably getting a slanted view ...

Frank, 55

The cautionary tone of the previous message was often repeated by participants who reported on 'others' who had made poor decisions about online information and/or who were at risk from online misinformation.

I expect that it is difficult for the average person to differentiate among objective, reliable sites for health information and those on the fringe, or that are simply trying to sell a product. That is more true for the less-educated and older seniors with little or no computer experience, who seem to believe that everything that comes from a computer must be true.

Laura, 63

Public policy and governance

Participants were often vehement in their discussion of policy issues related to health care for seniors. A recurring topic was the high cost of health care for older Americans.

Health care for seniors needs to be fixed! People on a fixed income do not need to be paying more for their healthcare than someone with a high-paying job; they need to be paying less.

Sherry, 56

Several respondents framed this concern for cost and policy in the larger context of the growing number of seniors and the fact that health care will become an even bigger problem as the baby boom generation ages.

I believe that this country has forgotten their senior citizens by cutting so much medical coverage and drug plans. We have contributed so much to this country and get so little; this is going to be worse for those behind us in age.

Tina, 60

The responses above reflect another related topic that emerged from the data. Many participants reported that the health care system is broken and needs to be fixed.

I believe there are significant improvements that must be made regarding health care issues for seniors even going as far as suggesting that the country explore socializing medicine in some form so that health care is available to all of our citizens.

April, 59

Several respondents commented on specific problems that they have identified with the Medicare system.

My largest healthcare issue is insurance and lack of coverage for certain things through Medicare. If Medicare doesn't pay, supplemental doesn't pay, such as for annual physical. It would appear to me that this is preventive health care and to cover this examination would make sense. ... I feel this needs to be confronted.

Erik, 66

These strong negative reactions also spread to other aspects of the 'business' of health care.

Insurance companies have too much control over health issues.

Paul, 70

I pay more now for medical procedures than before as my employer is shifting more of the medical burden to me, so would like to use the internet to become a better shopper for medical care and procedures. Right now it is nearly impossible to find what things cost in hospitals, doctors, etc., for what are essentially routine medical procedures such as colonoscopies, upper endoscopies, etc. Hopefully in time the internet will change such that I will be able to find the information I need to become a better medical shopper as far as costs go.

Rita, 65

Prescription drugs

The topic of drugs and pharmaceutical companies elicited vehement responses from participants and cost was often a central concern.

Prescription drug costs are criminally high. Seniors without adequate private medical insurance have a difficult time coping with the expense. The new federal Medicare plan for drugs is far too complicated and largely inadequate.

Bob, 59

Concerns about prescription drugs extended beyond Medicare coverage for pharmaceuticals. Respondents were also often critical of the business practices of pharmaceutical companies – particularly their advertising strategies.

I think the advertising of new meds to the general public is nuts, as well as humorous as to potential side effects. Only a hypochondriac or someone who thinks he/she is smarter than their doctor would want to tell their doctor what meds they should take or what new medical condition they have, which condition a pharma company has just created as the illness of the week, e.g., restless leg syndrome.

Rick, 59

Participants often reflected on the potential negative impacts that these commercial interests were having on Internet health communication.

Entirely too many web sites that are supposed to offer medical information are nothing more than poorly disguised commercials.

Nancy, 57

Many participants suggested that pharmaceutical companies offer little of value in online health communication because they are less interested in honest communication and more interested in gaining new customers. Interestingly, however, 37 per cent of all seniors who have ever gone online have sought information on prescription drugs (Rideout *et al.* 2005); perhaps skepticism sometimes succumbs to curiosity.

Pharmaceutical companies may have conflicts of interest issues when discussing medical issues and promoting their latest products as cures.

Rachel, 71

I do not trust Big Pharma Co's. I believe they lie for profit and take advantage of the American people (elderly especially). Doctors have some good knowledge but always lean toward Big Pharma.

Don, 59

Deferment to doctors

Even though many participants indicated that they value the medical information that they are able to find online (despite some frustrations noted in earlier comments), many reported that they balance this information very carefully with what they receive from medical professionals.

I trust my family doctor and specialists far more than I do the internet. I do research health topics on the net but carefully consider the source when evaluating validity.

Melissa, 59

In fact, many respondents seem to use Internet information to help them prepare for a visit to the doctor.

I think that properly designed research on the internet can provide the layman with tremendous knowledge and insights before going to a doctor to seek treatment. It calms the patient and provides for informed decision making, as well as communicating with the doctor in a more direct and forthright manner.

Donna, 65

These comments suggest that some participants view the Internet as part of a medical system that is basically 'whole.' While they sometimes wish their doctors would pay more attention to patient-driven information and also wish that they had more face-to-face time with doctors, many participants evaluated the overall health system as serving them well, while also often recognizing that they were 'blessed' to have such good relationships with doctors.

I have an excellent physician, who takes all the time I want to discuss my aches and pains and together we decide what course of action is best. I know I can call him at any time with my concerns, reactions to medications, etc. Everyone should be so blessed!

Joyce, 57

Actively managing their own health

As noted in the previous section, many respondents felt that the health care system was serving them well. But many other participants expressed frustration with the health care system – a frustration that often led them to feel that they were isolated in their health concerns rather than partnering with medical professionals.

> I find it hard to go to the doctor often enough and getting through to his office or him or even his nurse to talk directly is very hard, always have to leave a message and they don't call back, sometimes in his office I forget all I need to talk to him about and it gets frustrating.
>
> Jessica, 55

To overcome frustrations with doctors, some respondents reported taking a very active role in their own health care. In fact, a strong theme emerged suggesting that the doctor/patient relationship has changed and that the ability to inform oneself using online health information sources helped to facilitate this change. But one of the first steps in making this evolving relationship work is the importance of taking an active role in evaluating the quality of online information.

> Internet medical sites, like any internet sites, can be reliable or not. It is up to the consumer to note the date a web page was last updated, and to consider whether the source of information is reliable or not.
>
> Tanya, 70

Armed with good information, many participants felt that they were empowered and sometimes obligated to take care of their own health.

> I do not believe physicians walk on water and they do make mistakes so it is still up to the individual patient to be informed and make decisions on their healthcare with the physician, not go along with everything especially if they do not feel comfortable with a physician recommendation.
>
> Linda, 68

As they manage their own health care, many respondents report that the Internet fills in a variety of 'gaps' that are left by the medical community.

> I think it's extremely important to be able to get accurate medical information on the internet, since physicians no longer answer any questions by phone and we cannot afford to go in very often as retirees.
>
> Lynn, age not disclosed

Social/lifestyle issues

An interesting phenomenon that emerged in many responses was that the participants in this study are often information providers for individuals within their social networks.

> I am fortunate to be in good health. I live in a senior community and very often my neighbors come to me to do research for them on the internet for health related information.
>
> Mary, 62

In fact, quite a few respondents reported that they personally had little need of the health care system. As noted in the previous quotes, this did not mean that they did not search for online health information. Rather, the combination of their overall healthiness and their technological capabilities often put them in a leadership position for communicating about health among their peer groups. Many of these respondents focused on the importance of healthiness, exercise, and wellness as part of the aging process.

> Frankly, I don't have health issues at all. I eat right and exercise regularly. If I did have problems, I'd consult my doctor, but I'd also probably look for detailed information on the internet to increase my knowledge about any problem. I'm sure the net is invaluable to people who have health issues, but I'm glad I'm not one of them.
>
> Felicia, 61

Some participants chose to comment on some aspects of online communication that are not always directly related to health care and health information seeking. In particular, there was a fairly large subcategory of comments that addressed the social aspects of online communication.

> The internet makes my life much easier by keeping me easily in touch with people at their convenience.
>
> John, 72

Several participants noted the unique opportunities for community building that are available because of the Internet.

> For those of us who are disabled and somewhat homebound, the internet provides our social interaction, information, recreation, opportunities for volunteerism, and the great sense that we are still part of the global community.
>
> Ken, 64

But comments about the social benefits of the Internet were often counter-balanced by concerns about potential negative social consequences.

> I believe that the internet, like most things, has both good and bad aspects. It can help one learn innumerable things, but it can also tend to isolate people who use the computer as a substitute for the outside world.
>
> Rachel, 71

Technological/information savvy

Finally, the brief profile of respondents provided earlier makes it clear that this is a fairly 'high end' sample of seniors. Some participants provided background on how they had acquired their technical skills. Many reported that they were surprised with the relative ease with which they were able to learn to find information online.

> I love being able to surf the internet and computers in general. I think more seniors should try learning about computers as, once you get involved, it is not as difficult as one might think. I have also learned that it is really hard to 'break' one.
>
> Todd, 60

Several of the participants reported learning to use technology when they were still employed. Those workplace uses carried over into their personal comfort with health information seeking behaviors after retirement.

> Though my husband and I are seniors now we have used a computer for the past 25 years in our professional work. We are both architects. But I do notice that some people of our age are afraid of using computers. They have no confidence because unlike the new generation they have not had the opportunity to use computers since grade school.
>
> Julie, 61

Other participants noted the need for senior-specific training in using computers and the Internet – particularly for health-related information.

> I feel there needs to be more training available for seniors to use the internet to research what their doctors tell them.
>
> Bonnie, 64

While many of the participants were savvy about technology, a few reported that they had found technology to be personally challenging.

> In my early computer days, I definitely felt like a square peg in a round hole. I'm slowly learning, its rough teaching old dogs new tricks. The computer is still formidable to me but amazing as well.
>
> Caroline, 64

Many of the participants suggested that technology challenges applied more to 'others' than to themselves. This applied both to the basic technology and to the ability to interpret health information effectively.

> The internet is a valuable resource for those able and knowledgeable in/about accessing it. For many my age that's likely a bit of a problem.
>
> Ellen, 68

Selective coding

In the third stage of coding, selective coding, three themes emerged as over-arching categories for the eight axial categories. These themes include empowerment, personal and professional communities, and watchdogs and peer assumptions; these themes will be discussed in turn while drawing upon relevant theory in health communication to inform the discussion.

Empowerment

Analysis revealed that members of this group of seniors are quite proactive and increasingly taking health care into their own hands through the use of health information on the Internet. Perhaps given the repeated distaste for and distrust of the government's handling of health care (especially related to Medicare), these seniors have been forced to seek alternatives to restore their perceived health care efficacy. Unable to count on 'the system' to protect them, older adults may perceive that the best course of action regarding health is to be their own keepers. Thus, the Internet may offer them a form of empowerment. Participants expressed a real desire for themselves and their peers to be increasingly proactive in their health care, and responses such as 'I make the final decision on whether I will follow a treatment or not,' 'many times I have been able to help myself without going to the doctor,' and 'seniors must take initiative and be aggressive in their care,' illustrate this empowerment. Some seniors even self-diagnosed their conditions when unable to afford diagnostic tests. Empowerment seems to stem from the perceived value of the Internet as a resource, the active role seniors are playing in their health care, and the technologically savvy nature of this sample of seniors, categories that emerged in axial coding; these three factors may be working in concert to yield an empowered group of senior health information consumers.

Cusack (1995: 307) posits 'empowerment means not giving power to people, but enabling them to exercise their power.' Thus, the Internet must not be conceptualized simply as an automatic entitlement of power to seniors using it for health information. Instead, scholarly research must reveal how to best enable them to exercise the potential power of the web in health care. It is not adequate to assume that its resources empower health information consumers; instead, research must determine *how* to empower older adult populations. The results in this chapter reveal a sense of empowerment among the participants. However, both a strength and a limitation of this study is that the population under investigation comprised current Internet users. The use of existing Internet users in this study allowed richer and more comprehensive themes and categories surrounding web use to emerge. These findings can and should guide future research to test their applicability to non-Internet users. Perhaps these themes and categories may be used to reveal barriers for non-adopters. Yet, as they were garnered from a group already more technologically disposed, these results may not be generalized to the entire population of seniors. Thus, the enabling of empowerment is critical in making broader groups of seniors active but critical consumers of health information on the Internet. The empowerment that is representative of this group of participants may provide such a model guiding research focusing on non-users of the Internet for health information.

Personal and professional community

Lack of access to quality health care information and providers may be an impetus for the empowerment of seniors using the Internet for health information. In a somewhat similar vein, the isolation from the health care system that seniors experience may be a driving force for them to create new communities on the Internet where they can seek support from others suffering from similar conditions as well as engage in dialog with friends and family. Fear of misinformation, public policy and governance, prescription drugs, deferment to doctors, and social/lifestyle issues are categories that emerged in axial coding and may collectively contribute to this need for community on the Internet for seniors. Participants' comments such as 'I believe the internet to be a very good companion for seniors who have little personal attention and are unable to research due to their personal health issues,' 'I particularly like sites where others like me can give their experiences and opinions on health related issues,' and 'for those of us who are disabled and somewhat home-bound, the internet provides our social interaction, information, recreation, opportunities for volunteerism and the great sense that we are still part of the global community' illustrate the need for both companionship and learning on the Internet. Likewise, the Kaiser Family Foundation survey revealed 'one of the intangible potential benefits of the internet is helping socially isolated seniors keep in touch with family and friends' (Rideout *et al.* 2005). The results of that study revealed that about one-third of online seniors consider email and the Internet a very important part of their life they would not want to do without, and more than half of online seniors in the study noted that email makes it easier to keep in touch with friends and family (Rideout *et al.* 2005).

Albrecht and Goldsmith (2003) note two areas in health communication research on the processes and effects of social support especially pressing for theory development: structural aspects such as networks and the transaction processes occurring therein. Communication in support relationships is critical to coping with health crises. This analysis reveals a very powerful and far-reaching network – the Internet – with great potential to provide support and coping for seniors. The heuristic value of this paper is realized in both of the promising avenues identified by Albrecht and Goldsmith (2003) in theory building. The presence of the Internet as a community health network is revealed at a most basic level with this research; future research should be conducted to illuminate the structure of what promises to be a complex yet important network for seniors on the web. Further, this research identifies the nature of dialog on the Internet for informational and other more social motivations among older adults using the Internet for health information. Future research can use this analysis and the categories and themes revealed therein to frame studies on the transactional nature of health communication among seniors on the Internet. Further, supportive communication, particularly in a health context, does not occur in isolation; instead, dyads and group settings are links in an overarching communication network. The Internet as a source of health information and dialog is a fascinating place to study these communicative networks as it provides both a community for support and coping as well as access to unlimited health resources.

Relative to other demographics, older patients face particular challenges with respect to adherence to health treatments and care regimens due to co-morbidity, and adherence remains a significant and much researched obstacle in treating older patients (Brown *et al.* 2003). Adherence enhancement is an important part of older patient–provider interaction research, which continually reveals that communication is the best predictor of seniors' adherence to health regimens (McLane *et al.* 1995). Given the critical role of communication, the Internet communities that seniors are creating may be an important area for improving their adherence to health care regimens. Research must continue to investigate how Internet networks can be used to enhance adherence; these peer networks may build communities in which physicians also participate. Given the accessibility and broad network of Internet communication dyads in cyberspace, this research presents exciting applied areas for stimulating the adherence and, ultimately, the health of older Americans.

Interaction on the Internet may be studied by applying health communication models such as the Roter Interaction Analysis System (RIAS) (for a review, see Roter & McNeilis 2003). Although RIAS is traditionally used to measure verbal exchange between patients and providers, a useful and applicable extension of the model could be used to examine Internet dialog among patients, providers, *and* peer groups. RIAS seems to be particularly salient to studying Internet health communities as it is derived from a social exchange orientation 'consistent with health education and empowerment perspectives that view the medical encounter as a meeting between experts and is grounded in an egalitarian model of patient–provider partnership that rejects expert domination and passive patient roles' (Roter & McNeilis 2003). Senior users of the Internet for health information and community may be practicing this egalitarian model as they assume active patient roles as well as seek and proffer advice through internet dialog.

Yet, this 'cyber community' on the Internet was not immune from criticism; one participant made the point that this Internet community fosters isolation and withdrawal from the 'real world.' Internet communities may create a safe haven for seniors, particularly those homebound or alienated from their health care providers. Thus, this is where the notion of empowerment is critical. Although seniors may benefit greatly from using the Internet for health information in areas such as adherence, it should not be used as a crutch replacing health care providers and human interaction.

Watchdogs and peer assumptions

The final theme emerging through selective coding was one in which seniors were adopting watchdog roles for their peers and making assumptions about others' use of the Internet. This category seemed to be one of the most cross-cutting to emerge in axial coding. The notion that 'others' should be cared for was present in comments that were coded in almost every category; yet, fear of misinformation, deferment to doctors, actively managing their own health, social/lifestyle issues, and technological/information savvy seemed to be the most relevant categories. Comments such as 'I guess I am more comfortable with the internet than many people my age' and 'I feel many seniors do not know enough to make informed decisions on their own … although I can make informed decisions myself' illustrated a sense of empowerment over their health care superior to that held by peers as well as assumptions of the vulnerability of the 'other.' Participants also offered suggestions such as 'seniors need direction as to good sites and questionable ones' that suggest a watchdog role. One participant said,

> I expect that it is difficult for the average person to differentiate among objective, reliable sites for health information and those on the fringe, or that are simply trying to sell a product. That is more true for the less-educated and older seniors with little or no computer experience, who seem to believe that everything that comes from a computer must be true.
>
> Laura, 63

The participants in this study who, as noted earlier, were fairly experienced Internet users, felt self-empowered while at the same time expressing concern for their peers who use the Internet for health information. Assuming this 'watchdog' role, participants made recommendations to help guide those less tech-savvy toward safe use of the Internet for health information. Theoretically, there seemed to be somewhat of a third-person effect occurring (Davison 1983, 1986). The well-grounded perceptual component of Davison's (1983) third-person effect posits that message recipients believe others are more easily influenced by persuasive messages than they are. Davison's (1983, 1986) germinal work on the third-person effect extends the perceptual component in order to make behavioral predictions that build on the perceptual component and predict that biased perceptions will result in action to mitigate the impact of the message on others. Therefore, the behavioral component of the third-person effect predicts that a message receiver will take some action to control for the perceived effects of a message on some other group when a perceptual bias occurs.

In the current application, the 'message' may be conceptualized as health information on the Internet. The results of this analysis indicate that seniors believe their peers are vulnerable to misinformation on the Internet. Thus, they enact these watchdog roles to account for the perceived bias in message reception. Future research could use the third-person effect as the theoretical framework from which to study seniors' consumption of health information on the Internet to disclose any behavioral implications of perceptual bias.

Limitations and future directions

Several limitations are important to note. First, as detailed in the method section, this is not a random sample of all older adults. Thus, it is not appropriate to generalize from the participants in this study to all older Americans. Future scholars may wish to further develop the ideas presented here into quantitative survey research and field that research among a representative sample of both users and non-users of the Internet. Such a study would need to identify ways to reach that sample that might include online surveys but would also provide other ways for users to respond that enable even non-Internet users to participate.

Additional qualitative research should explore the findings of this study in more depth. Those future studies might benefit from narrowing, rather than widening, the participant group. For example, it could be important to identify why some seniors adopt a watchdog role and specific factors inducing their peer assumptions. 'Watchdog seniors' – most likely the earliest of adopters – may be powerful tools in diffusing health information and proper use of health information on the web to peers who are slower or reticent to adopt.

Conclusion

This study sought to gain insight into the use of the Internet for health information by those who are in an older demographic group and who are Internet users. In particular, the researchers sought to discover how these seniors view this digital environment as a resource for health information. The results of this analysis indicate that the Internet is a source of empowerment and community. Yet, perceived disparities exist among seniors regarding their peers' ability to take advantage of the powerful resource for health communication and information.

Clearly, seniors are not granted equal or automatic access to the Internet; older adults who are well-off financially, educated and male are more likely to have access (Meischke *et al.* 2005). Knowledge gaps and socioeconomic barriers may prevent access. Failure to critically consume information may place others at risk of misinformation. The results of this study suggest that participants recognized the tremendous potential of the Internet as a resource for health information. Yet, scholarly research must identify how to enable empowerment among broader senior audiences. Meischke *et al.* (2005) recognize that, given the disparity in access and difficulty of use of the Internet for many senior adults, it is imperative for health professionals to reveal new ways in which the Internet can be used more effectively to reach more seniors.

Doctors – those health professionals in most frequent contact with these audiences – are not encouraging older patients to use the Internet for health information seeking or communication. Less than 10 per cent of seniors reported that their physicians had ever inquired about whether the senior had Internet access, and less than 3 per cent of seniors have ever had a doctor recommend a particular health or medical website to them (Rideout *et al.* 2005). Further scholarly research must reveal important communicative networks within dyads on the Internet to find out how to better facilitate communication among those using it for health information, ultimately enriching adherence to health regimens and practice. Self-empowerment gleaned through Internet access and use may also manifest in better perceived health. Meischke *et al.* (2005) found a positive correlation between perceived general health and access to the Internet among seniors, as those with more access reported better health.

This study revealed many powerful categories and themes surrounding Internet use in senior health care. These themes are likely to grow in importance as baby boomers age and the demands on the health care systems that serve seniors increase.

Notes

1 The online panel is an opt-in, informed consent, privacy-protected 'subject pool' for web-based research. Panelists are recruited from around the world through collaborative agreements with high traffic websites and online marketing efforts. Prospective panelists can learn about the panel by visiting http://adresearch.advertising. utexas.edu/survey/online_panel/main.html.

Bibliography

6, P., Leat, D., Steltzer, K. & Stoker, G. (2002) *Toward holistic governance: the new reform agenda*, Basingstoke: Palgrave.

24dash (2007) *Telecare is the 'key' to future of social care in UK*. Available from http://www.24dash.com/health/27204.htm (accessed 1 December 2007).

Albrecht, T.L. & Goldsmith, D.J. (2003) 'Social support, social networks, and health', in T.L. Thompson, A.M. Dorsey, K.I. Miller & R. Parrott (eds) *Handbook of health communication*, Mahwah, NJ: Lawrence Erlbaum, pp. 263–84.

Antaki, C. & Widdicombe, S. (1998) *Identities in talk*, London: Sage Publications.

Appadurai, A. (1986) 'Commodities and the politics of value', in A. Appadurai (ed.) *The social life of things: commodities in cultural perspective*, Cambridge: Cambridge University Press.

Arber, S. & Ginn, J. (eds) (1995) *Connecting gender and ageing: a sociological approach*, Buckingham: Open University Press.

Arksey, H., Jackson, K., Croucher, K., Weatherly, H., Golder, S., Hare, P., Newbronner, E. & Baldwin, S. (2004) *Review of respite services and short-term breaks for carers for people with dementia*, London: NHS SDO.

Askham, J. (1998) 'Supporting caregivers of older people: an overview of problems and priorities', *Australasian Journal on Ageing* 17: 5–7.

Atkinson, J.M. & Heritage, J. (1984) *Structures of social action*, Cambridge: Cambridge University Press.

Audit Commission (2004a) *Older people: a changing approach. Independence and well-being*. Available from http://www.audit-commission.gov.uk/reports

—— (2004b) *Implementing telecare: strategic analysis and guidelines for policy makers, commissioners and providers*. Available from http://www.audit-commission.gov.uk/olderpeople (accessed 14 August 2008).

—— (2004c) *Assistive technology: independence and well-being*. Available from http://www.audit-commission.gov.uk/olderpeople (accessed 14 August 2008).

Austin, J.L. (1962) *How to do things with words*, New York: Oxford University Press.

AXA (2007) *Global retirement scope*. Available from http://www.axa.co.uk/media/pressreleases/2007/pr20070202_1100.html (accessed 24 May 2006).

Baines, S., Gannon-Leary, P. & Walsh, S. (2004) 'Framework for Multi-Agency Environments (FAME): final report of the learning and evaluation', Newcastle upon Tyne: The Newcastle Centre for Social and Business Informatics, University of Newcastle upon Tyne. Available from http://www.fame-uk.org/archive/strand/downloads/decemberReport.pdf (accessed 3 January 2008).

Ballinger, C. & Payne, S. (2002) 'The construction of the risk of falling among and by older people', *Ageing and Society* 22: 305–24.

Bank, A.L., Arguelles, S., Rubert, M.P., Eisdorfer, C. & Czaja, S.J. (2006) 'The value of telephone support groups among ethnically diverse caregivers of persons with dementia', *The Gerontologist* 46: 134–38.

Barlow, J. & Breeze, M. (2005) *Teleshopping for people with limited mobility*, York: Joseph Rowntree Foundation.

Barlow, J., Bayer, S., Castleton, B. & Curry, R. (2005) 'Meeting government objectives for telecare in moving from local implementation to mainstream services', *Journal of Telemedicine and Telecare* 11: 49–51.

Barlow, J., Bayer, S. & Curry, R. (2006) 'Implementing complex innovations in fluid multi-stakeholder environments: experiences of "telecare"', *Technovation* 26: 396–406.

Barlow, J., Singh, D., Bayer, S. & Curry, R. (2007) 'A systematic review of the benefits of home telecare for frail elderly people and those with long-term conditions', *Journal of Telemedicine and Telecare* 13: 172–79.

Bass, D.M., McClendon, M.J., Brennan, P.F. & McCarthy, C. (1998) 'The buffering effect of a computer support network on caregiver strain', *Journal of Aging and Health* 10: 20–43.

Basting, A.D. (1998) *The stages of age: performing age in contemporary American culture*, Ann Arbor, MI: University of Michigan Press.

Berg, M. & Goorman, E. (1999) 'The contextual nature of medical information', *International Journal of Medical Informatics* 56(1/3): 51–60.

Beynon-Davies, P. & Lloyd-Williams, M. (1999) 'When health information systems fail', *Topics in Health Information Management* 20(1): 66–79.

Bijker, W.E. (1995) *Of bicycles, bakelites and bulbs: toward a theory of sociotechnical change*, Cambridge, MA: MIT Press.

Birren, J.E., Kenyon, G.M., Ruth, J.-E., Schroots, J.J.F. & Svensson, T. (eds) (1996) *Aging and biography. Explorations in adult development*, New York: Springer.

Borup, M., Brown, N., Konrad, K. & van Lente, H. (eds) (2006) 'Special issue on the sociology of expectations', *Technology Analysis and Strategic Management* 18(3/4): 285–98.

Bowers, S. (2007) 'NHS director general of IT quits after repeated system delays', *The Guardian* 18 June 2007. Available from http://www.guardian.co.uk/business/2007/jun/18/health.politics (accessed 14 August 2007).

Bowes, A. & McColgan, G. (2002) *Pilot evaluation of 'opening doors for older people' in 'wired' West Lothian – report to West Lothian Council*, Stirling: Department of Applied Social Science, University of Stirling.

—— (2003) *Evaluation of Home Comforts Smart Home Technologies Initiative – Final report to South Ayrshire Council*, Stirling: Department of Applied Social Science, University of Stirling.

Bowker, G. & Star, S.L. (1999) *Sorting things out: classification and its consequences*, Cambridge, MA: MIT Press.

Bradbury, R. (1995) *The illustrated man*, London: Harper Voyager.

Brennan, P.F., Moore, S.M. & Smyth, K.A. (1995) 'The effects of a special computer network on caregivers of persons with Alzheimer's disease', *Nursing Research* 44: 166–72.

Brink, P. (1986) 'Editorial: on the patient career', *West J Nurs Res* 8(1): 5–7.

Brown, J.B., Stewart, M. & Ryan, B.L. (2003) 'Outcomes of patient–provider interaction', in T.L. Thompson, A.M. Dorsey, K.I. Miller & R. Parrott (eds) *Handbook of health communication*, Mahwah, NJ: Lawrence Erlbaum, pp. 141–62.

Brown, N. & Bury, M. (2001) 'Illness narratives: fact or fiction?', *Sociology of Health and Illness* 23: 263–85.

Brownsell, G. (2000) 'Using telecare: the experiences and expectations of older people', *Generations Review* 10: 1–12.

Brownsell, S. & Bradley, D. (2003) *Assistive technology and telecare: forging solutions for independent living*, Bristol: Policy Press.

Brownsell, S. & Hawley, M. (2004) 'Fall detectors: do they work or reduce the fear of falling?', *Housing, Care and Support* 7: 18–24.

Brownsell, S., Aldred, H. & Hawley, M. (2006a) 'Telemonitoring chronic heart failure: interim findings from a pilot study in South Yorkshire', *The British Journal of Healthcare Computing & Information Management* 23(8): 14–18.

Brownsell, S., Blackburn, S., Aldred, H. & Porteus, J. (2006b) 'Implementing telecare: practical experiences', *Housing Care and Support* 9(2): 6–12.

Burchell, K. (2007) 'Empiricist selves and contingent "others": the performative function of the discourse of scientists working in conditions of controversy', *Public Understanding of Science* 16(2): 145–62.

Burrows, R., Nettleton, S., Pleace, N., Loader, B. & Muncer, S. (2000) 'Virtual community care? Social policy and the emergence of computer mediated social support', *Information, Communication & Society* 3(1): 28–37.

Bury, M. (2001) 'Illness narratives, fact or fiction?', *Sociology of Health and Illness* 21 (3): 263–85

Butler, J.P. (1990) *Gender trouble (thinking gender)*, New York: Routledge.

—— (1993) *Bodies that matter: on the discursive limits of 'sex'*, New York: Routledge.

—— (1997) *Excitable speech: politics of the performative*, New York: Routledge.

Carers UK (2007) *Real change, not short change-time to deliver for carers*, London: Carers UK.

Carnell, D. (2001) 'Boost to NHS information systems as NHS signs Microsoft deal', *British Medical Journal* 323: 1386 (15 December).

Casper, G.R., Calvitti, A., Brennan, P.F. & Overholt, J.L. (1995) 'ComputerLink: the impact of a computer network on Alzheimer's caregivers' decision-making confidence and skill', *Medinfo* 8: 1546.

Castells, M. (2000) *The rise of the network society*, 2nd edn, Oxford: Blackwell.

Centre for Policy on Ageing (2007) 'Single assessment process: national SAP resource'. Available from http://www.cpa.org.uk/sap/sap_about.html (accessed January 2008).

Challis, D., Stewart, K., Donnelly, M., Weiner, K. & Hughes, J. (2006) 'Care management for older people: does integration make a difference?', *Journal of Interprofessional Care* 20(4): 335–48.

Change Agent Team, Department of Health (2004) 'Changing times: improving services for older people'. Report on the work of the Health and Social Care Change Agent Team, 2003/04. London: Department of Health. Available from Commission for Social Care Inspection's Annual Report to Parliament, 'The state of social care in England 2006–7'.

Chen, Y. & Persons, A. (2002) 'Internet use among young and older adults: relation to psychological well-being', *Educational Gerontology* 28(9): 731–44.

Clark, H., Gough, H. & Macfarlane, A. (2004) *'It pays dividends': direct payments and older people*, Bristol: Policy Press.

Cohen, C. (2001) 'Guiding seniors', *RN* 64: 50–52.

Cohen, C., Teresi, J. & Blum, C. (1994) 'The role of caregiver social networks in Alzheimer's disease', *Social Science and Medicine* 38: 1483–90.

Commission for Social Care Inspection (2008) 'Annual Report to Parliament, "The State of Social Care in England 2006-07"'. Available from http://www.csci.org.uk/about_us/publications/state_of_social_care_07.aspx (accessed 10 December 2007).

Connecting for Health website available from http://www.cfh.nhs.uk (accessed January 2008).

Cooke, D.D., McNally, L., Mulligan, K.T., Harrison, M.J. & Newman, S.P. (2001) 'Psychosocial interventions for caregivers of people with dementia: a systematic review', *Aging and Mental Health* 5: 120–35.

Coope, B., Ballard, C., Saad, K., Patel, K., Bentham, P., Bannister, C., Graham, C. & Wilcock, G. (1995) 'The prevalence of depression in the carers of dementia sufferers', *International Journal of Geriatric Psychiatry* 10: 237–42.

Corbin, J.M. & Strauss, A.L. (1990) 'Grounded theory research: procedures, canons, and evaluative criteria', *Qualitative Sociology* 13: 3–19.

Cowan, D. & Turner-Smith, A. (1999) 'The role of assistive technology in alternative models of care for older people', in I. Sutherland (ed.) *With respect to old age: long term care – rights and responsibilities*, London: The Stationery Office.

Crang, M. & Graham, S. (2007) 'Sentient cities: ambient intelligence and the politics of urban space', *Information, Communication & Society* 10(6): 789–817.

Csikszentmihalyi, M. & Rochberg-Halton, E. (1981) *The meaning of things. Domestic symbols and the self*, Cambridge: Cambridge University Press.

Cusack, S.A. (1995) 'Developing a lifelong learning program: empowering seniors as leaders in lifelong learning', *Educational Gerontology* 21: 305–20.

Czaja, S.J. & Rubert, M.P. (2002) 'Telecommunications technology as an aid to family caregivers of persons with dementia', *Psychosomatic Medicine* 64: 469–76.

Davis, P. & Brown, M. (2007) *Community resource team overview. Provided services*, London: Hackney Borough Council.

Davison, W.P. (1983) 'The third-person effect in communication', *Public Opinion Quarterly* 47: 1–15.

—— (1986) 'The third-person effect revisited', *International Journal of Public Opinion Research* 8: 113–19.

Dawson, S., Slote Morris, Z., Erickson, W. Lister, G., Altringer, B., Garside, P. & Craig, M. (2007) *Engaging with care – a vision for the health and care workforce of England*, Nuffield Trust.

DeBakey, M.E. (1995) 'Telemedicine has now come of age', *Telemedicine Journal* 1 (1): 2–3.

Dent, M. (2002) *Managing professional identities: knowledge, performativities and the 'new' professional*, Routledge.

Dent, M. & Whitehead, S. (2002) 'Introduction: Configuring the "new" professional', in M. Dent & S. Whitehead (eds) *Managing professional identities: knowledge, performativities and the 'new' professional*, London: Routledge.

Department of Health (1998) *Information for Health: an information strategy for the modern NHS 1998–2005*, Leeds: NHS Executive.

—— (1999) *Our healthier nation saving lives*, London: The Stationery Office.

—— (2001a) *National service framework for older people – executive summary*. Available from http://www.dh.gov.uk/en/Publicationsandstatistics/Publications/PublicationsPolicyAndGuidance/DH_4010161 (accessed 24 May 2006).

—— (2001b) *Information for social care: a framework for improving quality in social care through better use of information and information technology*, London: Department of Health.

—— (2002a) *Information strategy for older people in England*, London: Department of Health.

—— (2002b) *Delivering 21st century IT support for the NHS: national strategic programme*, London: Department of Health. Available from www.doh.gov.uk/ipu/whatnew/deliveringit/index.htm

—— (2002c) *Fair access to care services: guidance on eligibility criteria for adult social care*, London: Department of Health.

—— (2003) *Every child matters: change for children*, London: Department of Health.

—— (2004a) *National service framework for children*, London: Department of Health.

—— (2004b) *Choosing health: making healthy choices easier*. Available from http://www.dh.gov.uk/en/Publicationsandstatistics/Publications/PublicationsPolicyAndGuidance/DH_4094550 (accessed 24 May 2006).

—— (2005a) *Building telecare in England*, London: Department of Health.

—— (2005b) *Independence, well-being and choice: our vision for the future of social care for adults in England*, Cmnd 6499, London: The Stationery Office.

—— (2006) *Our health, our care, our say: making it happen*, London: NHS. Available from http://www.dh.gov.uk/Publicationsandstatistics/Publications/PublicationsPolicyAndGuidance/DH_4139925 (accessed 7 December 2007).

—— (2007a) *Putting people first: a shared vision and commitment to the transformation of adult social care*, London: Department of Health.

—— (2007b) 'World class commissioning. Vision summary'. Available at http://www.dh.gov.uk/prod_consum_dh/idcplg?IdcService = GET_FILE&dID = 155367&Rendition = Web (accessed 7 December 2007).

DH/ADASS/LGA/NHS (2007) 'Putting people first: a shared vision and commitment to the transformation of adult social care'. Available at http://www.dh.gov.uk/en/Publicationsandstatistics/Publications/PublicationsPolicyAndGuidance/DH_081118 (accessed December 2007).

Department of Trade and Industry (2000) *Health care 2020*, London: DTI.

Dewsbury, G., Rouncefield, M., Clarke, K. & Sommerville, I. (2004) 'Depending on digital design: extending inclusivity', *Housing Studies* 1(5): 811–25.

Dickinson, A. (2006) 'Implementing the single assessment process: opportunities and challenges', *Journal of Interprofessional Care* 20(4): 365–79.

Domènech, M., López, D., Callen, B. & Tirado, F.J. (2006) 'Elder people and artefacts: a problem of intimacy'. Paper presented at the EASST Conference, August 2006: 'Reviewing humanness: bodies, technologies and spaces', University of Lausanne, Switzerland.

Doughty, K. & Williams, G. (2001) 'Towards a complete home monitoring system'. Paper presented at the Royal Society for the Prevention of Accidents Conference on Safety in the Home, Stratford-upon-Avon, 12–13 November.

Doughty, K., Cameron, K.H. & Garner, P. (1996) 'Three generations of telecare of the elderly', *Journal of Telemedicine and Telecare* 2: 71–80.

Down, K. (2005) 'Anxiety grows over lack of critical debate', *The Guardian* G2 Social Care insert, 19 October, p. 4.

Ducatel, K. (2000) 'Ubiquitous computing: the new industrial challenge', in *The IPTS Report* 38: 16–21, Seville: IPTS Publications.

Dutton, W. & Helsper, E.J. (2007) *The Internet in Britain: 2007*, Oxford: Oxford Internet Institute, University of Oxford.

Edwards, D. (1991) 'Categories are for talking: on the cognitive and discursive bases of categorization', *Theory & Psychology* 1(4): 515–42.

Eisdorfer, C., Czaja, S.J., Loewenstein, D.A., Rubert, M.P., Argüelles, S., Mitrani, V.B. & Szapocznik, J. (2003) 'The effect of a family therapy and technology-based intervention on caregiver depression', *The Gerontologist* 43: 521–31.

Emery, D. (2001) 'Telecare in practice: a telecare initiative focusing on carers of older people based on ACTION', *Journal of Telemedicine and Telecare* 7: 41–8.

Emery, D., Hayes, B.J. & Cowan, A.M. (2002) 'Telecare delivery of health and social care', *Health Informatics Journal*, 8:1, 29–33.

Evers, S., Paulus, A. & Boonen, A. (2001) 'Integrated care across borders: possibilities and complexities', *International Journal of Integrated Care* serial online Sept 1: 1. Available from http://www.ijic.org/ (accessed 12 January 2008).

Eysenbach, G., Powell, J., Englesakis, M., Rizo, C. & Stern, A. (2004) 'Health related virtual communities and electronic support groups: systematic review of the effects of online peer interactions', *British Medical Journal* 328: 1166–70.

Faircloth, C.A., Boylstein, C., Rittman, M., Young, M.E. & Gubrium, J. (2004) 'Sudden illness and biographical flow in narratives of stroke recovery', *Sociology of Health and Illness* 26: 242–61.

FAME (2006) Framework for multi-agency environments webpage. Available from http://www.fame-uk.org (accessed 22 January 2008).

Featherstone, M. (1995) 'Post-bodies, ageing and virtual reality', reprinted in D. Bell & B. Kennedy (eds) (2000) *The Cybercultures Reader*, London: Routledge, pp. 609–18.

Ferri, C.P., Prince, M., Brayne, C., Brodaty, H., Fratiglioni, L., Ganguli, M., Hall, K., Hasegawa, K., Hendrie, H., Huang, Y., Jorm, A., Mathers, C., Menezes, P.R., Rimmer, E. & Scazufca, M. (2005) 'Alzheimer's Disease International. Global prevalence of dementia: a Delphi consensus study', *Lancet* 366: 2112–17.

Finkel, S., Czaja, S.J., Schulz, R., Martinovich, Z., Harris, C. & Pezzuto, D. (2007) 'E-care: a telecommunications technology intervention for family caregivers of dementia patients', *American Journal of Geriatric Psychiatry* 15: 443–48.

Fisher, P. (2007) 'Experiential knowledge challenges "normality" and individualised citizenship: towards "another way of being"', *Disability and Society* 22(3): 283–98.

Fisk, M.J. (1989) 'Telecare at home: factors influencing technology choices and user acceptance', *Journal of Telemedicine and Telecare* 4(2): 80–3.

—— (2003) *Social alarms to telecare: older people's services in transition*, Bristol: Policy Press.

Flynn, K.E., Smith, M.A. & Freese, J. (2006) 'When do older adults turn to the internet for health information? Findings from the Wisconsin longitudinal study', *JGIM: Journal of General Internal Medicine* 21: 1295–301.

Foucault, M. (1975) *The birth of the clinic: an archaeology of medical perception*, New York: Vintage Books.

Fox, S. (2006) *Online health search 2006*. Pew Internet & American Life Project. Available from http://www.pewinternet.org/pdfs/PIP_Online_Health_2006.pdf (accessed 10 July 2008).

Fox, S. & Rainie, L. (2002) *Vital decisions: how internet users decide what information to trust when they or their loved ones are sick*. Pew Internet & American Life Project. Available from http://www.pewinternet.org (accessed 10 July 2008).

Fox, S. & Fallows, D. (2003) *Internet health resources: health searches and email have become more commonplace, but there is room for improvement in searches and overall internet access*. Pew Internet & American Life Project. Available from http://www.pewinternet.org/pdfs/PIP_Health_Report_July_2003.pdf (accessed 10 July 2008).

Fox, S. & Madden, M. (2005) *Generations online*. Pew Internet & American Life Project. Available from http://www.pewinternet.org/pdfs/PIP_Generations_Memo.pdf (accessed 10 July 2008).

Gann, D., Burley, R., Curry, D., Phippen, P., Porteus, J., Wells, O. & Williams, M. (2000) *Healthcare and smart housing technologies*, Brighton: Pavilion Publishing Ltd.

Gannon-Leary, P., Baines, S. & Wilson, R. (2006) 'Collaboration and partnership: a review and reflections on a national project to join up local services in England', *Journal of Interprofessional Care* 20(6): 665–74.

Gilbert, G.N. & Mulkay, M. (1984) 'Scientists' discourse as a topic', in G.N. Gilbert and M. Mulkey, *Opening Pandora's Box: a sociological analysis of scientists' discourse*, Cambridge: Cambridge University Press.

Glasby, J. (2004) 'Social services and the single assessment process: early warning signs?', *Journal of Interprofessional Care* 18(2): 129–39.

—— (2007) *Understanding health and social care*, Bristol: Policy Press.

Glendinning, C., Powell, M. & Rummery, K. (eds) (2002) *Partnerships, New Labour and the governance of welfare*, Bristol: Policy Press, pp. 130–45.

Glueckauf, R.L. & Loomis, J.S. (2003) 'Alzheimer's caregiver support online: lessons learned, initial findings and future directions', *Neurorehabilitation* 18: 135–46.

Glueckauf, R.L., Ketterson, T.U., Loomis, J.S. & Dages, P. (2004) 'Online support and education for dementia caregivers: overview, utilization, and initial program evaluation', *Telemedicine Journal and E-Health* 10: 223–32.

Graham, S. & Wood, D. (2003) 'Digitizing surveillance: categorization, space, inequality', *Critical Social Policy* 23: 227–48.

Gullette, M.M. (2004) *Aged by culture*, Chicago, IL: University of Chicago Press.

Hailey, D., Roine, R. & Ohinmaa, A. (2002) 'Systematic review of evidence for the benefits of telemedicine', *Journal of Telemedicine and Telecare* 8 (Suppl 1, S1): 1–7.

Hardey, M. (2004) 'Internet et société: reconfigurations du patient et de la médecine?', *Sciences Sociales et Santé* 22(1): 21–42.

Hanson, J. & Osipovič, D. (2007) 'Making sense of sensors: interactions between older people and telecare devices within an extra care setting', 35th Annual Scientific Meeting of the British Society of Gerontology, Sheffield, UK.

Hanson, J., Osipovič, D., Hine, N., Amaral, T., Curry, R. & Barlow, J. (2007a) 'Lifestyle monitoring as a predictive tool in telecare', *Journal of Telecare and Telemedicine* 13 (Suppl 1): 26–8.

Hanson, J., Percival, J., Aldred, H., Brownsell, S. & Hawley, M. (2007b) 'Attitudes to telecare among older people, professional care workers and informal carers: a preventative strategy or crisis management?', *Universal Access in the Information Society* 6(2): 193–205.

Heath, H.B.M. & Watson, R. (2005) *Older people: assessment for health and social care*, Age Concern Books.

Heaton, J., Noyes, J., Sloper, P. & Shah, R. (2005) 'Families' experiences of caring for technology-dependent children: a temporal perspective', *Health and Social Care in the Community* 13(5): 441–50.

Hesse, B.W., Moser, R.P., Rutten, L.J.F. & Kreps, G.L. (2006) 'The Health Information National Trends Survey: research from the baseline', *Journal of Health Communication* 11: vii–xvi.

Hibbert, D., Mair, F.S., Angus, R.M., May, C., Boland, A., Haycox, A., Roberts, C., Shiels, C. & Capewell, S. (2003) 'Lessons from the implementation of a home telecare service', *Journal of Telemedicine and Telecare* 9 (Suppl 1, S1): 55–6.

HM Treasury (2002) 'The role of the voluntary and community sector in service delivery – a cross cutting review'. Available at http://www.hm-treasury.gov.uk/spending_review/spend_ccr/spend_ccr_voluntary/ccr_voluntary_report.cfm (accessed 7 December 2007).

Hobson-West, P. (2007) '"Trusting blindly can be the biggest risk of all": organised resistance to childhood vaccination in the UK', *Sociology of Health and Illness* 29: 198–215.

Holstein, R.C. & Lundberg, G.D. (2003) 'Letter to the editor: use of the internet for health information and communication', *JAMA: The Journal of the American Medical Association* 290: 2255–59.

Hopper, R. (1992) Telephone conversation, Bloomington, IN: Indiana University Press.

Hudson, B. (2002) 'Interprofessionality in health and social care: the Achilles' heel of partnership?', *Journal of Interprofessional Care* 16(1): 7–17.

Hughes, K. (2004) 'Health as individual responsibility. Possibilities and personal struggle', in P. Tovey, G. Easthorpe and J. Adams (eds) *The mainstreaming of complementary and alternative medicine, studies in social context*, London: Routledge, pp. 25–49.

Hutchby, I. (2001) *Conversation and technology: from the telephone to the internet*, Cambridge: Polity Press.

Hutchby, I. & Wooffitt, R. (1998) *Conversation analysis: principles, practices and applications*, Cambridge: Polity Press

Hyden, L.C. (1997) 'Illness and narrative', *Sociology of Health and Illness* 19: 48–69.

Imrie, R. (2003) 'Housing quality and the provision of accessible homes', *Housing Studies* 18: 387–408.

Jones, R.L. (2006) '"Older people" talking as if they are not older people: positioning theory as an explanation', *Journal of Aging Studies* 20: 79–91.

Kaufman, D.R. & Rockoff, M.L. (2006) 'Increasing access to online information about health: a program for inner-city elders in community-based organizations', *Generations* 30: 55–57.

Kaufman, S.R. (1986) *The ageless self, sources of meaning in late life*, Madison, WI: The University of Wisconsin Press.

Kerfoot, D. (2002) *Managing the professional man. Managing professional identities. Knowledge, performativity and the 'new' professional*, London and New York: Routledge, pp. 81–95.

King, N. (2004) *Assistive technology in extra care housing*, Housing Learning & Improvement Network Factsheet no. 5. London: Care Services Improvement Partnership, Department of Health.

King's Fund (2006) *Wanless social care review background paper: telecare and older people*, London: King's Fund.

Kleinman, A. (1988) *The illness narratives. Suffering, healing and the human condition*, New York: Basic Books.

Knapp, M. & Prince, M. (2007) on behalf of the Personal Social Services Research Unit, London School of Economics and the Institute of Psychiatry. *Dementia UK: A report into the prevalence and cost of dementia*, London: Alzheimer's Society.

Lancet (1995) 'Telemedicine: fad or future?', *The Lancet* 345: 73–74.

Larner, A.J. (2003) 'Use of the internet and of the NHS Direct telephone helpline for medical information by a cognitive function clinic population', *International Journal of Geriatric Psychiatry* 18: 118–22.

Latour, B. (1987) *Science in action: how to follow scientists and engineers through society*, Cambridge, MA: Harvard University Press.

—— (2005) *Reassembling the social. An introduction to actornetworktheory*, Oxford: Oxford University Press.

Laviolette, P. & Hanson, J. (2007) 'Home is where the heart stopped: panopticism, chronic disease and housing telecare in Barnsley, UK', *Home Cultures* 3(3): 25–44.

Leadbeater, C. (2004) *Personalisation through participation: a new script for public services*, London: Demos.

Levin, E. (1997) *Carers: problems, strains and services*, Oxford: Oxford University Press.

Levy, S., Jack, N., Bradley, D., Morison, M. & Swanston, M. (2003) 'Perspectives on telecare: the client view', *Journal of Telemedicine and Telecare* 9: 156–60.

Lewis, J. (2001) 'Older people and the health–social care boundary in the UK: half a century of hidden policy conflict', *Social Policy and Administration* 35(4): 343–59.

Lie, M. & Sørensen, K (eds) (1996) *Making technology our own? Domesticating technology into everyday life*, Oslo: Scandinavian University Press.

Ling, T. (2002) 'Delivering joined-up government in the UK: dimensions, issues and problems', *Public Administration* 80(4): 615–42.

Lipskey, M. (1980) *Street-level bureaucracy*, New York: Russell Sage.

Livingstone, G.E., Manela, M. & Katona, C. (1996) 'Depression and other psychiatric morbidity in carers of elderly people living at home', *British Medical Journal* 312: 153–56.

Llewellyn, G., Balandin, S., Dew, A. & McConnell, D. (2004) 'Promoting healthy, productive ageing: plan early, plan well', *Journal of Intellectual & Developmental Disability* 29: 366–69.

Loader, B.D. (1998) 'Welfare direct: the emergence of a self-service welfare state?', in J. Carter (ed.) *Postmodernity and the fragmentation of welfare*, London: Routledge.

—— (1999) 'Informational health networks: health care organisation in the information age', in M. Purdy and D. Banks (eds) *Health and exclusion: policy and practice in health provision*, London: Routledge.

Lorig, K. (2002) 'Partnerships between expert patients and physicians', *The Lancet* 359: 814–15.

Loxley, J. (2006) *Performativity*, Abingdon, New York: Routledge.

Lupton, D. (1996) '"Your life in their hands": trust in the medical encounter', in V. James and J. Gabe (eds) *Health and the sociology of emotions*, Oxford: Blackwell, pp. 157–72.

Lyall, J. (2005) 'Balance of risk for telecare', *The Guardian* G2 Social Care insert, 19 October, p. 4.

Lymbery, M. (2006) 'United we stand? Partnership working in health and social care and the role of social work in services for older people, 2006', *British Journal of Social Work* 36: 1119–34.

Lyon, D. (2001) *Surveillance society*, Buckingham: Open University Press.

—— (2003) *Surveillance as social sorting: privacy, risk, and digital discrimination*, London: Routledge.

Lyotard, J.-F. (1984) *The postmodern condition: a report on knowledge* (Theory and History of Literature). University of Minnesota Press.

Macias, W. & McMillan, S.J. (2008) 'The return of the house call: the role of internet-based interactivity in bringing health information home to older adults', *Health Communication* 23(1): 1–11.

McCarthy, J. & Wright, P. (2004) *Technology as experience*, London: Sage Publications.

MacKenzie, D. (1998) 'The certainty trough', in R. Williams, W. Faulkner & J. Fleck (eds) *Exploring expertise*, Basingstoke: Macmillan, pp. 325–29.

Magnusson, L. & Hanson, E.J. (2003) 'Ethical issues arising from a research, technology and development project to support frail older people and their family carers at home', *Housing and Social Care in the Community* 11: 431–39.

Magnusson, L., Hanson, E. & Borg, M. (2004) 'A literature review study of information and communication technology as a support for frail older people living at home and their family carers', *Technology and Disability* 16: 223–35.

Mahoney, D.F., Tarlow, B.J., Jones, R.N., Tennstedt, S. & Kasten, L. (2001) 'Factors affecting the use of a telephone-based intervention for caregivers of people with Alzheimer's disease', *Journal of Telemedicine and Telecare* 7: 139–48.

Mahoney, D.F., Tarlow, B.J. & Jones, R.N. (2003) 'Effects of an automated telephone support system on caregiver burden and anxiety: findings from the REACH for TLC intervention study', *The Gerontologist* 43: 556–67.

Marwick, C. (1999) 'Cyberinformation for seniors', *Journal of the American Medical Association* 281: 1474–77.

Marziali, E. & Donahue, P. (2006) 'Caring for others: internet video-conferencing group intervention for family caregivers of older adults with neurodegenerative disease', *The Gerontologist* 46: 398–403.

Marziali, E., Damianakis, T. & Donahue, P. (2006) 'Internet-based clinical services: virtual support groups for family caregivers', *Journal of Technology in Human Services* 24: 39–54.

May, C., Allison, G., Chapple, A., Chew-Graham C., Dixon, C, Gask, L. Graham, R., Rogers, A. & Roland, M. (2004) 'Framing the doctor–patient relationship in chronic illness: a comparative study of general practitioners' accounts', *Sociology of Health and Illness* 26: 135–58.

May, C., Finch, T., Mair, F. & Mort, M. (2005) 'Towards a wireless patient: chronic illness, scarce care and technological innovation in the United Kingdom', *Social Science & Medicine* 61: 1485–94

McClendon, M.J., Bass, D.M., Brennan, P.F. & McCarthy, C. (1998) 'A computer network for Alzheimer's caregivers and use of support group services', *Journal of Mental Health and Aging* 4: 403–20.

McCreadie, C. & Tinker, A. (2005) 'The acceptability of assistive technology to older people', *Ageing & Society* 25: 91–110.

McGarry, J. & Arthur, A. (2001) 'Informal caring in late life: a qualitative study of the experiences of older carers', *Journal of Advanced Nursing* 33: 182–9.

McLane, C.G., Zyzanski, S.J. & Flocke, S.A. (1995) 'Factors associated with medication noncompliance in rural elderly hypertensive patients', *American Journal of Hypertension* 8: 206–9.

McLaughlin, J, Rosen, P., Skinner, D. & Webster, A. (1999) *Valuing technology: organisation, culture and change*, London: Routledge.

McMillan, S.J. & Macias, W. (forthcoming) 'Strengthening the safety net for online seniors: factors influencing differences in health information seeking among older internet users', *Journal of Health Communication*.

Mehnert, B. & Gardner, K. (1998) 'Seniors cruise the net for health information. NIH releases study showing older Americans don't want to be left behind on information superhighway', *NIH News Release*. Available from http://www.nih.gov/new/pr/dec98/nlm-04.htm (accessed 27 August 2007).

Meischke, H., Eisenberg, M., Rowe, S. & Cagle, A. (2005) 'Do older adults use the internet for information on heart attacks? Results from a survey of seniors in King County, Washington', *Heart & Lung* 34: 3–12.

Melzer, D., Hopkins, S., Pencheon, D., Brayne, C. & Williams, R. (1994) 'Dementia', in A. Stevens and J. Raftery (eds) *Health care needs assessment. The epidemiologically based needs assessment reviews*, Vol. 2, Oxford: Radcliffe Medical Press.

Monk, A. & Reed, D.J. (2007) 'Telephone conferences for fun: experimentation in people's homes'. Paper presented at the HOIT 07.

Moran, R. (1993) *The electronic home: social and spatial aspects*. Dublin: European Foundation for the Improvement of Living and Working Conditions.

Morrell, R.W. (2002) *Older adults, health information, and the world wide web*, Mahwah, NJ: Lawrence Erlbaum Associates, Inc.

Mort, M., May, C.R. & Williams, T. (2003) 'Remote doctors and absent patients: acting at a distance in telemedicine?', *Science, Technology, & Human Values* 28(2): 274–95.

Mort, M., Finch, T. & May, C.R. (2008) 'Making and unmaking telepatients', *Science, Technology and Human Values* 33 (forthcoming).

National Audit Office (2006) *Annual report 2006: helping the nation spend wisely*. Available from http://www.nao.org.uk/publications/annual06/nao_ar2006.pdf (accessed 24 May 2006).

National Service Framework for Older People (2001) London: Department of Health. Available from http://www.dh.gov.uk/En/Publicationsandstatistics/Publications/PublicationsPolicyAndGuidance/DH_4003066 (accessed 18 January 2008).

Newman, J. (2001) *Modernising governance: New Labour, policy and society*, London: Sage.

NHS Connecting for Health (2006) 'A National Framework for Electronic SAP implementation'. Available from http://www.cpa.org.ukysapye-sapyCFH-eSAPyIntro_Presentation_re_eSAP_(2).ppt (accessed 24 January 2008).

NHS Executive (1998) *Information for health. An information strategy for the modern NHS 1998–2005*, Leeds: NHS Executive.

NHS Information Authority (2004) *Making IT happen*, Brochure 1501, London: Department of Health.

Nielsen, J. (1993) *Usability engineering*, Boston, MA: AP Publishing.

Nies, H. & Berman, P. (eds) 'Integrating services for older people: a resource book for managers', European Health Management Association.

Nikander, P. (2000) '"Old" vs. "little girl": a discursive approach to age categorization and morality', *Journal of Aging Studies* 14(4): 335–58.

—— (2002) *Age in action. Membership work and stage of life categories in talk*, Helsinki: Finnish Academy of Science and Letters.

Norman, C.D. & Skinner, H.A. (2006) 'e-health literacy: essential skills for consumer health in a networked world', *Journal of Medical Internet Research* 8: e9. Available from http://www.jmir.org/2006/2/e9/ (accessed 3 February 2007).

Osipovič, D. & Hanson, J. (2007) 'The double life of the fall detector: older people's attitudes towards caring technology', Third International Conference on Technology, Knowledge and Society, New Hall College, Cambridge, 9–12 January 2007.

Oudshoorn, N. (2008) 'Diagnosis at a distance: the invisible work of patients and healthcare professionals in cardiac telemonitoring technology', *Sociology of Health & Illness* 30: 272–88.

Oudshoorn, N. & Pinch, T. (eds) (2003) *How users matter. The co-construction of users and technology*, Cambridge, MA, and London: MIT Press.

—— (2005) *How users matter: the co-construction of users and technology*. Cambridge, MA: MIT Press.

Pagnell, M., Spence, L. & Moore, R. (2000) *The market potential for smart homes*, York: Joseph Rowntree Foundation.

Parry, I. & Thompson, L. (1993) *Effective sheltered housing: a handbook*, London: Longman.

Parsons, T. (1951) *The social system*, New York: Free Press.

Payne, S., Kerr, C., Hawker, S., Hardey, M., & Powell, J. (2002) 'The communication of information about older people between health and social care practitioners', *Age and Ageing* 31: 107–17.

Payton, F.C., Brennan, P.F. & Silvers, J.B. (1995) 'Cost justification of a community health information network: the computerlink for AD caregivers', *Proceedings of the Annual Symposium on Computer Applications in Medical Care* 566–70.

Percival, J. & Hanson, J. (2006) 'Big brother or brave new world? Telecare and its implications for older people's independence and social inclusion', *Critical Social Policy* 26(4): 888–909.

Philip, I. (2007) *A recipe for care – not a single ingredient. Clinical case for change: report*, London: Department of Health.

Phillipson, C. (1998) *Reconstructing old age. New agendas in social theory and practice*, London: Sage Publications.

Pickering, A. (1995) *The mangle of practice: time, agency and science*, Chicago, IL: Chicago University Press.

Pilling, D., Barrett, P. & Floyd, M. (2004) *Disabled people and the internet: experiences, barriers and opportunities*, York: Joseph Rowntree Foundation.

Porteus, J. & Brownsell, S. (2000) *Using telecare: exploring technologies for independent living for older people*, London: Anchor Trust.

Postle, K. (2002) 'Working "between the idea and the reality": ambiguities and tensions in care managers' work', *British Journal of Social Work* 32: 335–1.

Potter, J. & Wetherell, M. (1987) *Discourse and social psychology: beyond attitudes and behaviour*, London: Sage.

Powell, J. & Clarke, A. (2007) 'Investigating internet use by mental health service users: interview study', *Studies in Health Technology and Informatics* 129: 1112–16.

Powell, J., Robison, J., Roberts H. and Thomas G. (2007) 'The single assessment process in primary care: older people's accounts of the process', *British Journal of Social Work* 37(6): 1043–58.

Powell, J., Chiu, T. & Eysenbach, G. (2008) 'Networked technologies supporting carers of people with dementia: systematic review', *Journal of Telemedicine and Telecare* 14: 114–16.

Pragnell, M., Spence, L. & Moore, R. (2000) *The market potential for smart homes*, York: Joseph Rowntree Foundation.

Prottas, J.M. (1979) *People processing: the street-level bureaucrat in public service bureaucracies*, Lexington, MA: D.C. Heath.

Pusey, H. & Richards, D. (2001) 'A systematic review of the effectiveness of psychosocial interventions for carers of people with dementia', *Aging and Mental Health* 5: 107–19.

Reed, D.J. (2001) '"Making conversation": sequential integrity and the local management of interaction on internet newsgroups'. Paper presented at the 34th Annual Hawaii International Conference on System Sciences (HICSS-34). Outrigger Wailea Resort, Maui.

—— (2003) 'Fun on the phone. The situated experience of recreational telephone conferences', in M. Blythe, A. Monk, K. Overbeeke & P. Wright (eds) *Funology. From usability to enjoyment*, London: Kluwer, pp. 67–80.

—— (2004) 'What recreational telephone conferencing can teach us about the future of mass communications', *Interactions*. Special issue on mass media, XI(2): 63–67.

—— (2004) 'The flow-test: a method for understanding the good conversation'. Paper presented at the Games and Social Networks: A workshop on multiplayer games, British HCI 2004.

Reed, D.J. & Ashmore, M. (2000) 'The naturally-occurring chat machine', *Journal of Media and Culture* 3(4).

Reed, D.J. & Monk, A. (2004) 'Using familiar technologies in unfamiliar ways: learning from the old about the new', *Universal Access in the Information Society (UAIS)*, Special issue on design principles to support older adults, 3(2): 114–21.

Reed, J., Cook, G., Childs, S. & McCormack, B. (2005) 'A literature review to explore integrated care for older people', *International Journal of Integrated Care* 5. Available from http://www.ijic.org/publish/issues/2005-1Arch/index.html?000208 (accessed 27 January 2008).

Rideout, V., Neuman, T., Kitchman, M. & Brodie, M. (2005) *E-health and the elderly: how seniors use the internet for health information*. Kaiser Family Foundation. Available from http://www.kff.org/entmedia/7223.cfm (accessed 10 July 2008).

Robinson, L., Hutchings, D., Corner, L., Finch, T., Hughes, J., Brittain, K. & Bond, J. (2007) 'Balancing rights and risks: conflicting perspectives in the management of wandering in dementia', *Health, Risk and Society* 9: 389–406.

Rogers, E.M. (1995) *Diffusion of innovations*, New York: Free Press.

Roine, R., Ohinmaa, A. and Hailey, D. (2001) 'Assessing telemedicine: a systematic review of the literature', *Canadian Medical Association Journal* 165(6): 765–71.

Roter, D. & McNeilis, K.S. (2003) 'The nature of the therapeutic relationship and the assessment of its discourse in routine medical visits', in T.L. Thompson, A.M. Dorsey, K.I. Miller & R. Parrott (eds) *Handbook of health communication*, Mahwah, NJ: Lawrence Erlbaum, pp. 121–40.

Royal Society (2006) *Digital healthcare: the impact of information and communication technologies on health and healthcare*, London: The Royal Society.

Ruth, J.-E. & Kenyon, G.M. (1996) 'Biography in adult development and aging', in J.E. Birren, G.M. Kenyon, J.-E. Ruth, J.J.F. Schroots & T. Svensson (eds) *Aging and biography. Explorations in adult development*, New York: Springer.

Saetnan, A. (2002) 'The co-construction of video surveillance and public spaces – a media snapshot'. Paper presented at the EASST 2002 Conference, University of York, UK.

Sävenstedt, S., Sandman, P.O. & Zingmark, K. (2006) 'The duality in using information and communication technology in elder care', *Journal of Advanced Nursing* 56: 17–25.

Secretary of State, Social Enterprise in Primary and Community Care (2006) Available from http://www.socialenterprise.org.uk/documents/socialenterprise_primary_community_care.pdf (accessed 12 January 2008).

Schechner, R. (1985) *Between theatre and anthropology*, University of Pennsylvania Press.

Schegloff, E.A. (1977) 'Identification and recognition in interactional openings', in I. de Sola Pool (ed) *The social impact of the telephone*, London and Cambridge, MA: MIT Press.

Schenkein, J. (1978) 'Sketch of an analytic mentality for the study of conversational interaction', in J. Schenkein (ed.) *Studies in the organisation of conversational interaction*, London: Academic Press.

Shilling, C. (1993) *The body and social theory*, London: Sage.

Seymore, W. & Lupton, D. (2004) 'Holding the line online: exploring wired relationships for people with disabilities', *Disability and Society* 17(4): 291–305.

Silverman, D. (1998) *Harvey Sacks. Social science & conversation analysis*. Cambridge: Polity Press.

Silverstone, R. & Hirsch, E. (eds) (1992) *Consuming technologies: media and information in domestic spaces*, London and New York: Routledge.

Sismondo, S. (2003) *An introduction to science and technology studies*, Malden, MA: Blackwell Publishing.

Sixsmith, A. & Sixsmith, J. (2000) 'Smart care technologies: meeting whose needs?', *Journal of Telemedicine and Telecare* 6(Suppl 1, S1): 190–92.

Smale, G., Tuson, G., Biehal, N. and Marsh, P. (1993) *Empowerment, assessment, care management and the skilled social worker*, London, The Stationery Office.

SSIA (2007) 'Joint working'. Available from http://www.ssiacymru.org.uk/index.cfm?articleid = 2206 (accessed 14 November 2007).

Star, S.L. (1999) 'The ethnography of infrastructure', *American Behavioral Scientist* 43 (3): 377–91.

Strauss, A.L. & Corbin, J.M. (1990) *Basics of qualitative research: grounded theory, procedures and techniques*, Newbury Park: Sage.

Stuck, A.F., Siu, A.L., Wieland, G.D., Adams, J. & Rubenstein, L.Z. (1993) 'Comprehensive geriatric assessment: a meta-analysis of controlled trials', *The Lancet* 342 (8878): 1032–36.

Suchman, L. (2002) 'Practice-based design of information systems: notes from the hyperdeveloped world', *Information Society* 18: 139–44.

Sugden, R., Wilson, R. & Cornford, J. (2008) 'Re-configuring the health supplier market: changing relationships in the primary care supplier market in England', *Health Informatics Journal* 14(2): 113–124.

Sutherland, S. (1999) *Royal Commission on long term care (1999) with respect to old age*, London: The Stationery Office.

Tang, P., Gann, D. & Curry, R. (2000) *Telecare: new ideas for care and support @ home*, Bristol: Policy Press.

Taylor, D. & Bury, M. (2007) 'Chronic illness, expert patients and care transition', *Sociology of Health and Illness* 29: 27–45.

Timmermans, S. & Berg, M. (2003) 'The practice of medical technology', *Sociology of Health & Illness* 25: 97–114.

TSA (Telecare Services Association) (2007) 'About telecare'. Available from http://www.Telecare.org.uk/information/42290/about_Telecare (accessed 1 December 2007).

Turner-Smith, A. (2000) 'Help required: what is assistive technology?', *The Newsletter of the Centre of Rehabilitation Engineering*, Review 17, Spring: 18–24.

UMEA Institute of Design (2006) 'Home diagnostics for the elderly patient', Umea University Working Paper, UMEA: Sweden.

Urry, J. (2000) *Sociology beyond societies*, London: Routledge.

Usabilitynews (2007) 'Telecare technology launched as demand for 'social inclusion' rises'. Available from http://www.uabilitynews.com/news/article3857.asp (accessed 1 December 2007).

Vanderheiden, G. & Iacona, S. (2001) 'Technologies for successful aging: information technology impacts', *Journal of Rehabilitation Research and Development* 38: S52–S53.

van Wijngaarden, J., de Bont, A. & Huijsman, R. (2006) 'Learning to cross boundaries: the integration of a health network to deliver seamless care', *Health Policy* 79(2–3): 203–13.

Virilio, P. (1998) *Polar inertia*, London: Sage.

Wan, T.T.H., Ma, A. & Lin, B.Y.J. (2001) 'Integration and the performance of healthcare networks: do integration strategies enhance efficiency, profitability, and image?', *International Journal of Integrated Care* Jun 1: 1. Available from http://www.ijic.org/ (accessed 27 January 2008).

Wanless, D. (2002) *Securing our future health: taking a long-term view*, London: HM Treasury. Available from http://www.hm-treasury.gov.uk/Consultations_and_Legislation/wanless/consult_ wanless_final.cfm (accessed 18 May 2006).

—— (2004) *Securing good health for the whole population*, London: HM Treasury.

Wathen, N., Wyatt, S. & Roma, R. (eds) (2008) *Health information and technology: mediating health information in a changing socio-technical landscape*, Basingstoke: Palgrave Macmillan.

Webster, A. (2002) 'Innovative health technologies and the social: redefining health, medicine and the body', *Current Sociology* 50(3): 443–57.

—— (2007) *Health, technology and society: a sociological critique*, Basingstoke: Palgrave Macmillan.

Webster, A. & Eriksson, L. (2008) 'Governance-by-standards in the field of stem cells: managing uncertainty in the world of "basic innovation"', *New Genetics and Society* (forthcoming).

Whitaker, R. (1999) *The end of privacy*, New York: New York Press.

White, M.H. & Dorman, S.M. (2000) 'Online support for caregivers. Analysis of an internet Alzheimer mailgroup', *Computers in Nursing* 18: 168–76.

Whitten, P. & Richardson, J. (2002) 'A scientific approach to the assessment of telemedicine acceptance', *Journal of Telemedicine and Telecare* 8: 246–48.

Wieck, K. (2001) *Making sense of the organization*, Thousand Oaks, CA: Sage.

Willis, S. L. (2006) 'Technology and learning in current and future generations of elders', *Generations* 30: 44–48.

Wilson, P.M. (2001) 'A policy analysis of the expert patient in the United Kingdom: self-care as an expression of pastoral power?', *Health and Social Care in the Community* 9(3): 134–42.

Wilson, R., Baines, S., Cornford, J. & Martin, M. (2007) '"Trying to do a jigsaw without the picture on the box": understanding the challenges of care integration in the context of single assessment for older people in England', *International Journal of Integrated Care* 7. Available from http://www.ijic.org/publish/articles/000288/article.pdf (accessed 12 January 2008).

Wolpert, H.A. & Anderson, B.J. (2001) 'Management of diabetes: are doctors framing the benefits from the wrong perspective?', *British Medical Journal* 323: 994–96.

Woolgar, S. (ed.) (2002) *Virtual society? Technology, cyberbole, reality*, Oxford: Oxford University Press.

Worth, A. (2001) 'Assessment of the needs of older people by district nurses and social workers: a changing culture?', *Journal of Interprofessional Care* 15(3): 257–66.

Yalom, I. (1995) 'The therapeutic factors in group psychotherapy', in I. Yalom (ed.) *Theory and practice of group psychotherapy*, New York: Basic Books.

Yin, R.K. (2003) *Case study research: design and methods*, London: Sage.

Index

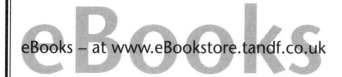